Cold Water Diving
A Guide to Ice Diving

SECOND EDITION

Cold Water Diving
A Guide to Ice Diving

SECOND EDITION

By John N. Heine

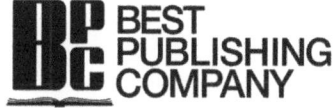

The opinions expressed in this work are those of the author and do not reflect the opinions of Best Publishing Company or its editors.

Information contained in this work has been obtained by Best Publishing Company from sources believed to be reliable. However, neither Best Publishing Company nor its author guarantees the accuracy or completeness of any information published herein, and neither Best Publishing Company nor its author shall be responsible for any errors, omissions, or claims for damages, including exemplary damages, arising out of use, inability to use, or with regard to the accuracy or sufficiency of the information contained in this publication.

The editor, author, publisher, or any other party associated with the production of this diving manual does not accept responsibility for any accident or injury resulting from the use of materials contained herein. Diving is an activity that has inherent risks. An individual may experience injury that can result in disability or death. All persons who wish to engage in diving activities must receive professional instructions. This diving manual does not constitute legal, medical, or other professional advice. Information in this publication is current as of the date of the printing.

All rights reserved. No part of this book may be reproduced, stored in a retrieval system, or transmitted in any form or by any means, electronic, mechanical, photocopying, recording, or otherwise, without written permission from the publisher.

Copyright © 2015 by Best Publishing Company

ISBN: 978-193-0536-87-6
Library of Congress Control Number: 2015950551

Best Publishing Company
631 US Highway 1, Suite 307
North Palm Beach, FL 33408

Table of Contents

Acknowledgments vii

Warning ix

Chapter 1: An Introduction to Diving 1
   Cold Water Diving 1
   History of Ice Diving 2
   Cold Water and Ice-Diving Environment 4
      Seasonal Thermal Stratification in Lakes 4
      Variation in Ocean Temperatures 4
      Freshwater Ice 8
      Lake Environments 9
      Rivers 10
      Sea Ice 10

Chapter 2: Training 13
   Classroom Curriculum 13
      Cold Weather Environment 14
      Cold Water Environment 14
      Equipment 14
      Ice-Diving Operations 14
      Dive Planning and Personnel 14
      The Dive 15
      Safety and Emergency Procedures 15
   Confined-Water Training 16
   Drysuit Training 16
   Suggested Drysuit Skills 16
   Ice Diving Open-Water Training 17

Chapter 3: Equipment for Ice Diving 21
   Thermal Protection for Divers 21
      Types of Drysuits 22
      Features of Drysuits 23
      Accessories 27
      Undergarments 29
      Weight and Buoyancy Systems 32
      Care and Maintenance 33
      Service and Repairs 34
   Cylinders and Valve Configurations 35
   Regulators 36
   Dive Knife, Mask, and Fins 37
   Instruments, Gauges, and Computers 38

| Dive Lights 38
        Surface-Supplied Diving 39
        Safety Harness and Lines 39
        Thermal Protection for Surface Personnel 42
        Emergency Equipment 42
        Additional Equipment 42

Chapter 4: Ice-Diving Operations 45
        Evaluating Ice Conditions 45
        Preparing the Site 46
        Dive Planning and Personnel 50
        Diving at Altitude 52
        Suiting Up 52
        The Dive 53

Chapter 5: Safety and Emergency Procedures 57
        Environmental Hazards 57
        Emergency Procedures 58
                Regulator Freeze Up 58
                Inflator Valve Malfunction 58
                Dropped or Lost Weight Belt 59
                Entanglement 59
                Flooded Drysuit 60
                Loss of the Dive Hole 60
                Wind Chill 62
                Frostbite 62
                Hypothermia 63
                Management of Heat-Loss Victims 64
                Conscious Diver with Lung Overpressure or Decompression Illness ... 65
                Unconscious Diver 66

Summary 69

References 71

Index 73

About the Author 79

Acknowledgments

This publication would not have been possible without the help of many people. Thanks to Dr. Jim McClintock for getting me to Antarctica the first three times to dive in some of the most spectacular under-ice areas of the world. Special thanks to the National Science Foundation Office (now Division) of Polar Programs and the various support contractors for providing excellent support of science and scientific diving in the Antarctic. Specifically, Jim Stewart, Rob Robbins, Steve Rupp, Jim Mastro, and Jeff Bozanic were instrumental in conducting a safe scientific diving program during my many years at McMurdo Station and Palmer Station in Antarctica.

I spent many enjoyable hours with Dr. John Oliver and the Benthic Bubs of the Moss Landing Marine Laboratories, diving in the Bering and Chukchi Seas near Alaska. That was my first real introduction to cold water diving. Bill Briggs and John Brooks of the National Park Service were extremely helpful during an ice-diving training course that they sponsored and I conducted.

I especially thank the people who have contributed photographs and technical information for this book: Margaret Amsler, Dale Andersen, John Brooks, Paul Dayton, Henry Kaiser, Neal Langerman, Jim Mastro, Frank Morrow, Rob Robbins, Steve Rupp, and Dale Stokes. All other photographs are by the author, unless noted otherwise.

I appreciate the assistance of Neal Langerman and Dale Andersen, who critiqued early drafts of the first edition.

Last, I thank my wife, Nisse, who is extremely tolerant and supportive of my projects, which often require considerable time away from home.

WARNING

Scuba diving is a potentially hazardous activity. Ice diving is a type of scuba diving that requires special equipment and training. This book is not a substitute for scuba diving or ice diving instruction. You must be certified for scuba diving and for diving in cold water and under ice before undertaking this type of activity.

Note: Some photographs in this book show untethered divers under the ice. This is a special case for scientific divers in the US Antarctic Program when conditions allow. All other under-ice dives must be tethered.

CHAPTER 1
An Introduction to Ice Diving

Cold water and ice diving can be extremely challenging yet rewarding experiences for the adventurous diver. Diving in these environments requires thoughtful planning, preparation, training, and the utmost dedication to safety. The rewards are many, including excellent visibility, a calm surface platform from which to work, a sense of accomplishment from performing an extreme challenge, and the enjoyment of being outdoors in cold weather.

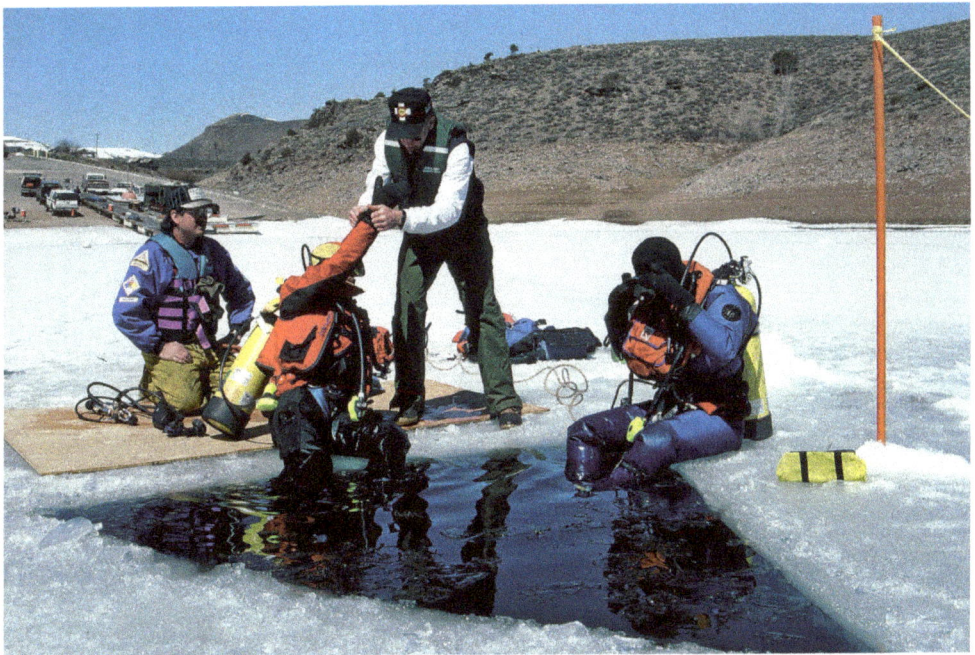

Fig. 1.1 — A well-organized ice-diving operation requires a surface support team for the divers. (Photo courtesy of John Brooks)

Cold Water Diving

Cold water diving is defined as diving in water temperatures below about 40°F (4.5°C). Many lakes and ocean regions have water temperatures this low in seasons other than winter. While this is not freezing water, it is sufficiently cold to require special thermal protection and regulator care. Hypothermia and equipment malfunction are special risks associated with cold water diving. Considerations for low surface temperatures, thermal stress, equipment malfunction, and logistics increase the complexity of this special type of diving.

Diving under ice is a special situation that increases the dive complexity by adding a ceiling overhead for divers. This requires a team of surface tenders and special procedures both to ensure that divers are able to return to the entry hole and to deal with any emergencies that might arise.

There are many things to consider when planning and executing a cold water dive. Training, site selection, equipment considerations, shelter, safety and emergency equipment, and personnel are all important. It takes considerable time to select and prepare a site, suit in and out of drysuits, and conduct the dive. The following chapters will cover these topics in detail.

History of Ice Diving

Ice diving traditionally has been limited by thermal protection, chiefly in exposure-suit technology. In the early 1900s, salvage divers in Iceland were stationed on vessels to render assistance to fishing boats whose nets became entangled. They used relatively crude commercial diving dress. With the advent of scuba equipment in the 1950s, the Icelandic Coast Guard began training personnel for open-sea diving operations, often in water temperatures that were near freezing.

In Antarctica, scientists began diving in ice-cold water for research in 1957, making initial test dives to determine the feasibility of using diving equipment in these harsh environmental conditions. They used wetsuits, drysuits, and double-hose regulators, making dives that lasted up to one hour. Custom-tailored wetsuits up to 3/8 inch (9 mm) thick reportedly worked well, especially if the diver kept swimming to generate body heat. The use of underwater floodlights enabled diving even in the dark months of the Antarctic winter. Divers, who were tethered for safety and communications reasons, wore wetsuits underneath drysuits with built-in mittens. While this combination proved extremely bulky, it allowed divers to remain under the ice for up to one hour. During these early southern polar dives, researchers documented the first observations of the abrasive action of ice in shallow subtidal areas.

In the mid-1950s, Canadian naval divers began Arctic diving operations for surveys. Research diving in cold marine water and freshwater began in the 1960s. In the Sub-Igloo expedition, an 8-foot (2.5-meter) transparent sphere was anchored to the sea floor in the Canadian Arctic to support divers underwater. It was found that human efficiency underwater could be enhanced by the presence of a rest station offering air and warmth.

More recently, ice diving has been associated with oil and gas development and mining activities. In the Arctic, a controlled oil spill experiment found that oil under the ice seeps up toward the surface of the ice through small hollow brine channels, which then freeze, essentially sandwiching the oil into the ice.

Naval oceanographers conducted early under-ice scuba dives in the Arctic region near Point Barrow, Alaska, to evaluate equipment, safety, and efficiency of dives in harsh, freezing conditions. They used two-stage double-hose primary regulators and various types of single-hose regulators as backups, wetsuits, and the first commercial drysuit, the Poseidon Unisuit.

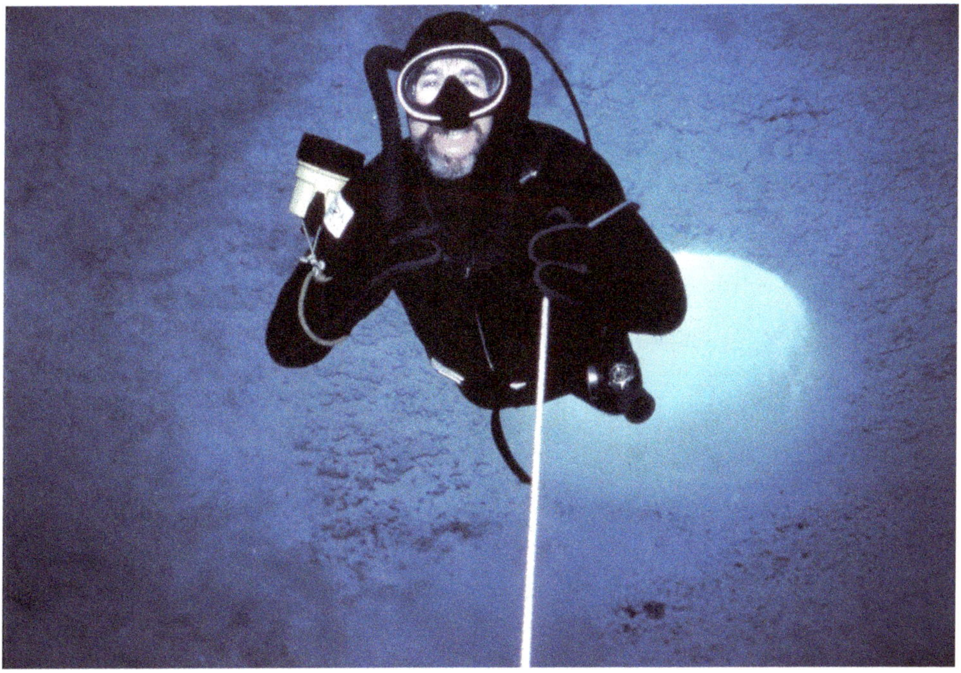

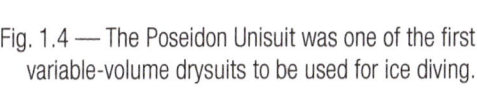

Fig. 1.2 — Early ice divers wore wetsuits and used double-hose regulators. (Photo courtesy of Paul Dayton)

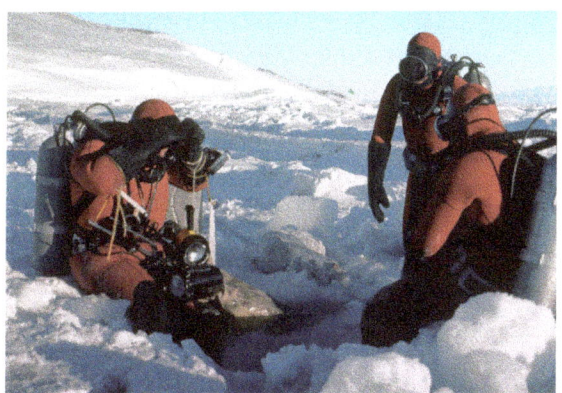

Fig. 1.3 — Pioneering scientific divers wore prototype drysuits in the Antarctic in the 1960s. (Photo courtesy of Paul Dayton)

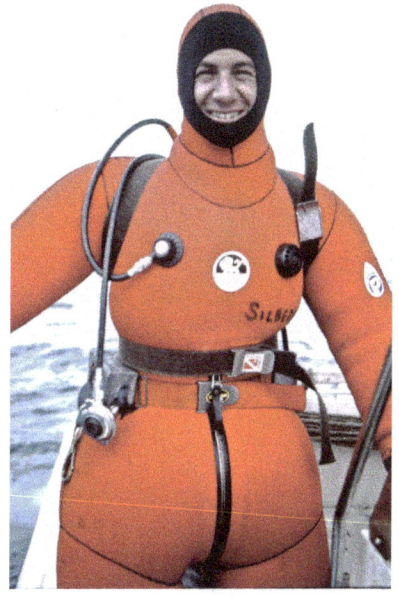

Fig. 1.4 — The Poseidon Unisuit was one of the first variable-volume drysuits to be used for ice diving.

The JIM suit, a one-atmosphere diving suit used primarily in commercial diving, was used in the Arctic on dives to 905 feet (272 m), where the water temperature was 27.5°F (-3°C). The suit is heated by the diver's body heat and CO_2 scrubbers, which stabilize the system at 70°F (21°C). This allowed an underwater time of 5 hours and 59 minutes on the dive.

Recreational ice diving has been practiced for decades but is becoming more popular with the advent of reasonably priced drysuits. Technical divers see this type of diving as a challenge and a way to keep diving in the winter in areas that experience freezing temperatures.

Cold Water and Ice-Diving Environment

Seasonal Thermal Stratification in Lakes

Lakes in the temperate zone have a general seasonal pattern of thermal stratification. During the summer months, the upper two meters of lake water will absorb more than one-half of the sun's radiation and will be warmed. A typical summer stratification has three distinct water layers. The *epilimnion* is the surface layer of warm water, typically 55°F (13°C) to 75°F (24°C), which reaches a depth of about 30-50 feet (10-15 m). Below this layer is a region of sharp decline in temperature, termed the *thermocline* or *metalimnion*. The temperature here can drop by as much as 30°F (15°C) in just a few meters of depth. The lowest layer of water is called the *hypolimnion*, which is a deep, cold, undisturbed layer of water that approaches the temperature of maximum density for freshwater: 39°F (4°C).

In the fall, as air temperatures begin to cool and the sun is not as high in the sky, the water cools to about 43°F (6°C), and wind-induced mixing of the water layers begins. This so-called fall turnover results in an isothermal condition in which the water temperature is about 39°F (4°C) from the surface to the bottom.

As winter ensues, further cooling of surface water occurs, and ice begins to form. A reverse stratification can occur in which colder (less dense) water overlies warmer (more dense) water.

In the spring, as ice melts and day length increases, the wind can induce a spring turnover that produces relatively isothermal water conditions of around 39°F (4°C). This is a general description of stratification in large temperate lakes, and many variations will be found due to climate, lake morphology, and movement of water masses.

Variation in Ocean Temperatures

Ocean surface layer temperatures can be extremely variable, depending upon factors such as latitude, climate, winds, and ocean currents. For example, at an open ocean station off the coast of Siberia, the water is at a uniform temperature of about 40°F (4.5°C) in March. The water continues to warm through the summer until reaching a typical maximum temperature of 60°F (15.5°C), and a marked thermocline develops, the depth of which depends on wind conditions. In the fall, as the surface water cools, it becomes denser and sinks. Winter conditions show uniform cold temperatures down to depths of 225 feet (70 m).

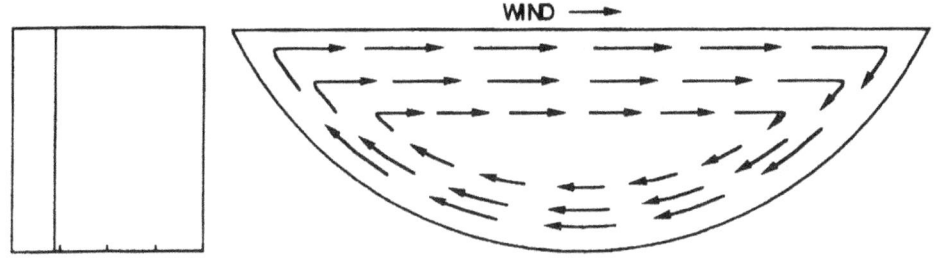
A. ISOTHERMAL WATER: SPRING OVERTURN

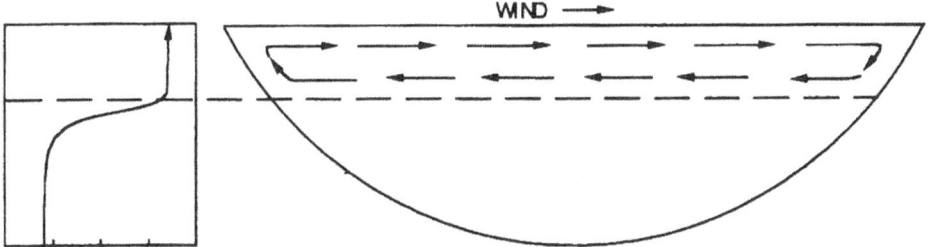
B. STRATIFIED WATER: SUMMER PERIOD

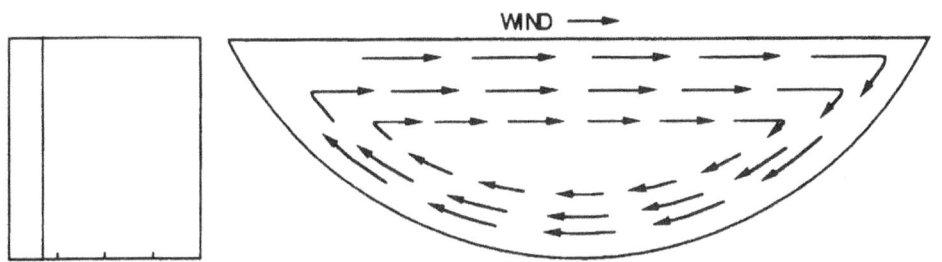
C. ISOTHERMAL WATER: FALL OVERTURN

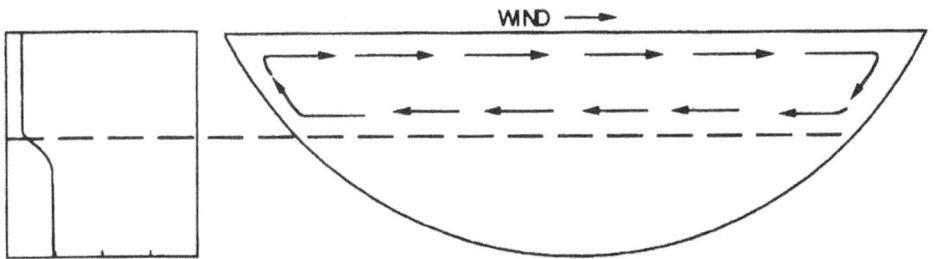
D. STRATIFIED WATER: WINTER PERIOD

Fig. 1.5 — The four seasons of lake stratification

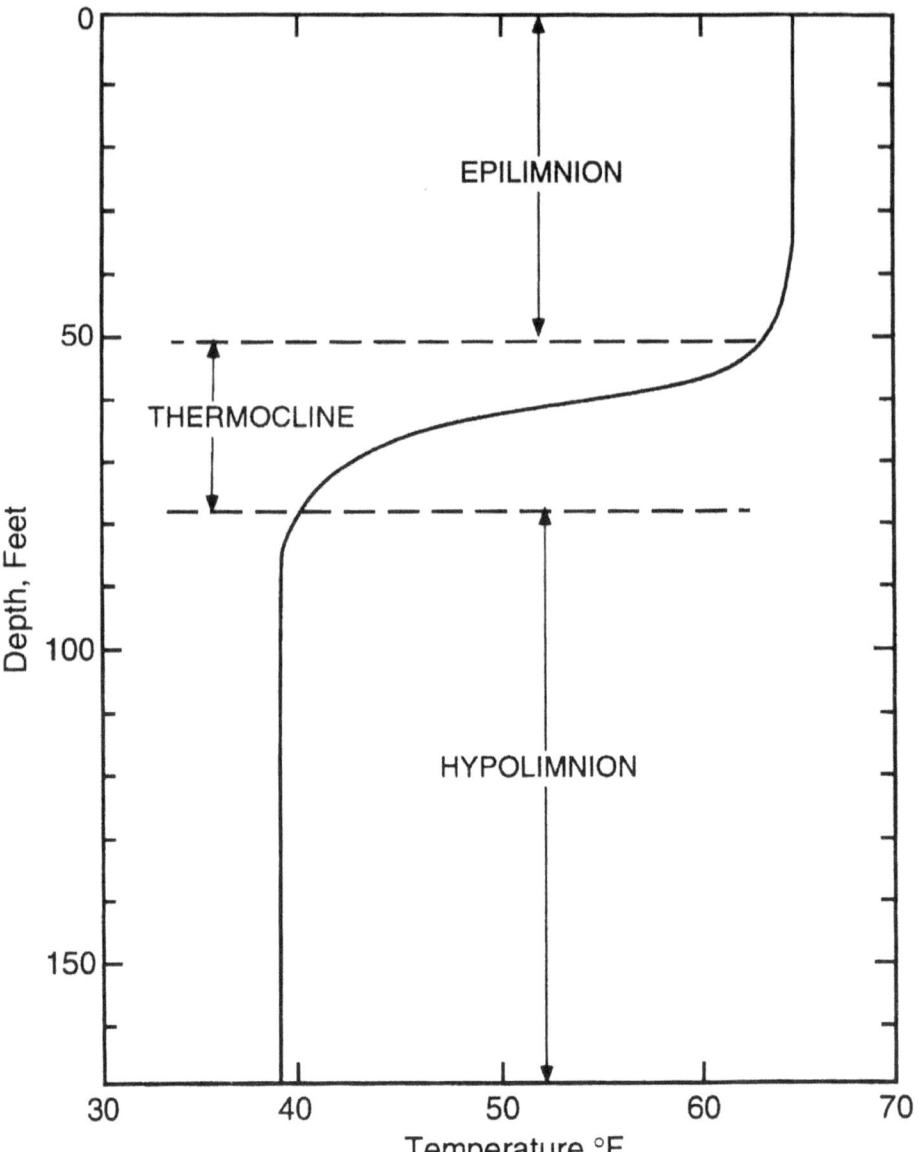

Fig. 1.6 — Lake water layer terminology

Other areas may show variations in ocean temperature that are related more to currents and wind patterns rather than to large changes in air temperature or available sunlight. In California, the prevailing current runs from north to south, bringing colder water along the coastline. Interestingly, the warmest water can be present in the winter, when the current typically runs south to north. In the spring, strong northwesterly winds cause upwelling, where surface waters are blown away from shore and replaced by deeper, cold water.

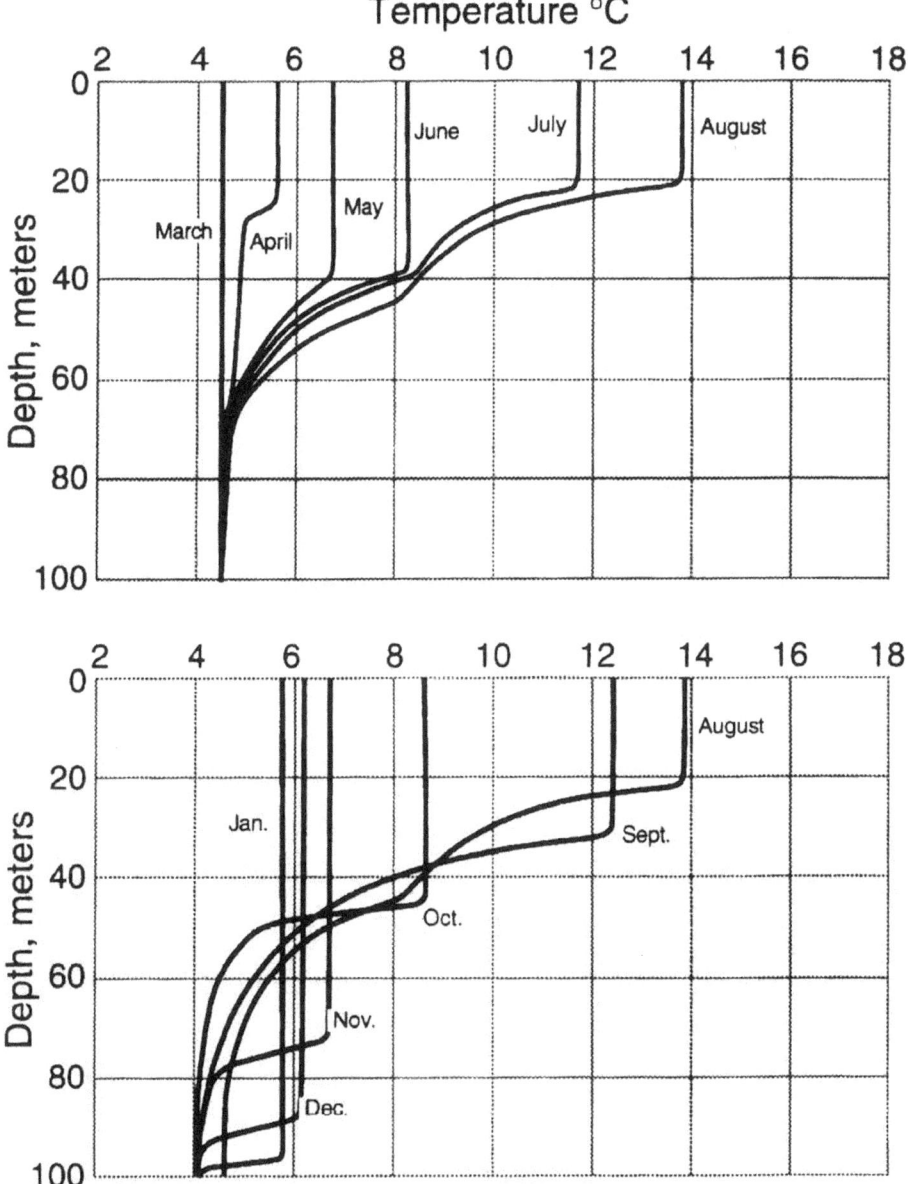

Fig. 1.7 — An example of the seasonal variation of ocean temperature in the North Pacific

On the East Coast of the United States, the Gulf Stream runs from south to north, bathing the coastline in relatively warm water. Northern states and eastern Canada experience winter freezing of the ocean waters due to the cold Labrador Current flowing from the north.

In the Arctic regions, new ice forms in the winter and melts during the following summer. In the Antarctic, the seasons are reversed. Although highly variable depending on the latitude and weather, new ice generally forms in the austral fall and winter (March–November) and melts in the austral summer (December–February).

Ice diving can be conducted in both freshwater and saltwater. The characteristics of ice, which are different for these two media, are discussed below. It is important for divers to have some knowledge of the physics behind ice formation, strength, and types of ice.

Freshwater Ice

Most liquids expand somewhat uniformly with increasing temperature. However, freshwater has a somewhat different pattern than other liquids. Between around 32-39°F (0-4°C), water contracts as the temperature increases. At 39°F (4°C), water has the least volume and maximum density. Pure water expands about 9% on freezing. This explains why ice floats and lakes freeze from the surface down.

Cold air temperatures cause the surface water to cool; when the water reaches 39°F (4°C), it becomes denser and sinks. This displaces warmer water up to the surface, which then becomes chilled. This continual mixing occurs, and the bottom water stays at a temperature of around 39°F (4°C), while the colder, less dense surface water freezes.

In North America, most alpine lakes and rivers north of about 35° north latitude usually have some ice cover each winter. Some large lakes, such as some of the Great Lakes, never form a complete ice cover due to strong winds blowing over a relatively deep body of water.

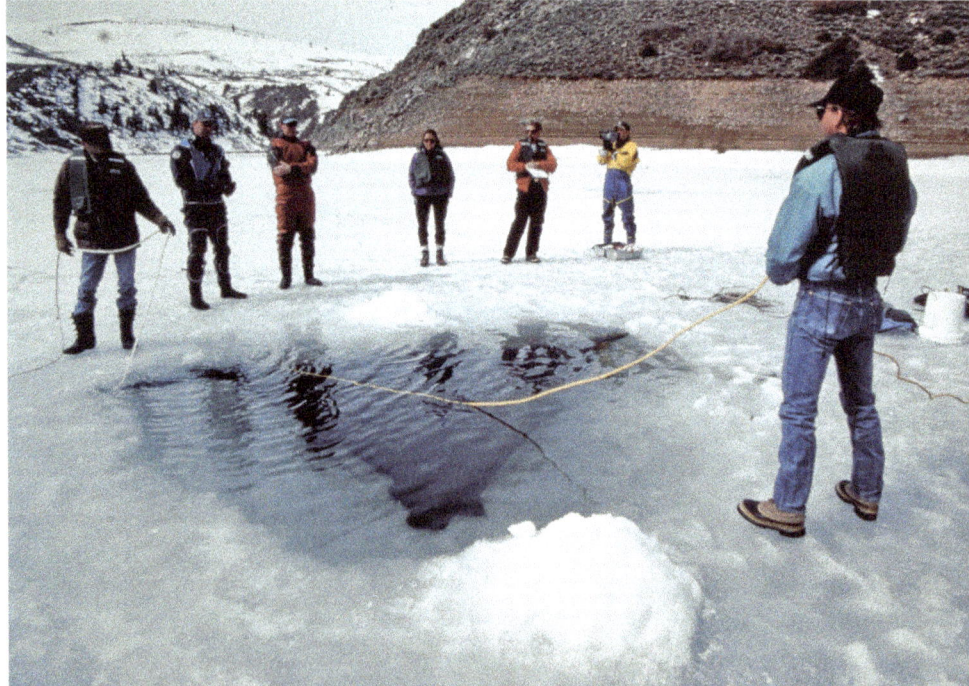

Fig. 1.8 — A freshwater lake in the mountains of Colorado freezes over in the winter.

This causes an upwelling of slightly warmer water to the surface, which delays the onset of freezing. However, a significant portion of the Great Lakes is covered with anywhere from 2 to 16 inches of ice during the winter. Underwater visibility under this ice can be as great as 100 feet in Lake Superior and remarkably lower in areas where there is significant runoff, nutrient enrichment, and fine sediment.

Terms used to describe freshwater ice are *clear ice*, which is nearly transparent, *bubbly ice*, which is translucent due to the trapped air bubbles, and *snow ice*, which is opaque or milky in appearance.

Lake Environments

Lakes vary tremendously with respect to water visibility, bottom terrain, thermoclines, and potential hazards. Many mountain lakes are clear, while lower-lying reservoirs or glacial lakes may be cloudy. The bottom terrain can consist of soft fine sediments that can be easily disturbed to rocky ledges of varying slopes.

There are potential hazards in some lakes and quarries that may impede a dive. Areas around dams or near roads may contain old cables, heavy equipment, fishing line, hooks, lures, and even automobiles. There is a possibility of encountering tree limbs or submerged structures. It is also possible for it to be quite dark under the ice.

If the lake is at altitude, the appropriate altitude dive tables, conversions, or dive computers must be utilized.

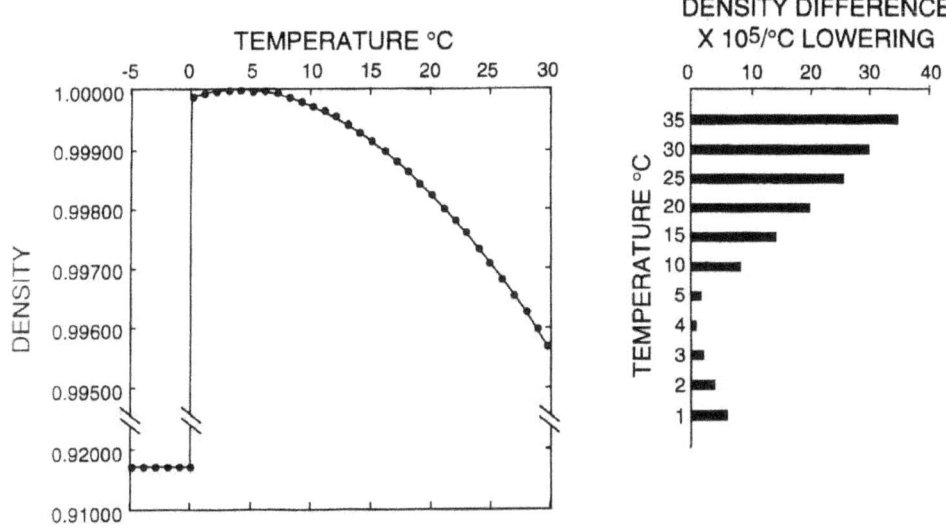

Fig. 1.9 — Freshwater has a unique pattern of density at different temperatures.

Rivers

Diving in cold or frozen rivers can be dangerous. No dive should be conducted under a frozen river where a current exists, as divers can be swept into areas where it is impossible to surface. Potential hazards underwater include tree limbs, sharp rocks, fishing line, hooks, lures, and nets.

Sea Ice

The low air temperature conditions of high latitude can cause the freezing of seawater. Normal salinity of seawater is 35 parts per thousand. This seawater will freeze at a temperature of 28.6°F (-1.9°C). As the water cools, small crystals called *frazil* begin to form. The dissolved solids are excluded from the frozen crystals so that sea ice has a much lower salinity than the surrounding water. A slushy mixture called *grease ice* develops and will form into a thin frozen sheet if conditions are calm. Wind and wave action can break these thin sheets into what is called *pancake ice*, which are small disks of ice about 1-3 feet (0.3-1m) in diameter. With further freezing, these disks can join together to form floes. Freezing generally continues from the bottom of the ice.

There are several types of sea ice. *Pack ice* forms seasonally in polar regions, moves with the wind and currents, and can be up to 6.5 feet (2 m) thick. It can be semipermanent above 75° latitude. When this ice collides together, breaks up, melts, and refreezes, the pack ice can take on a rough and jagged appearance. This is sometimes called *multiyear ice* because of its age and can be up to 12-20 feet (4-6 m) thick. *Polar ice*, which is permanent ice, can be more than 165 feet (50 m) thick. *Fast ice* is solid ice that is connected to the shoreline. It develops in the winter, disappears in the summer, and is usually about 6 feet (2 m) thick. This ice sheet continues to grow from the underside by the freezing of platelet ice crystals. These types of sea ice rarely exceed 13 feet (4 m) in thickness.

The small amount of salt in sea ice is concentrated in pockets of brine, forming brine channels, which are like underwater pinnacles hanging below the ice surface.

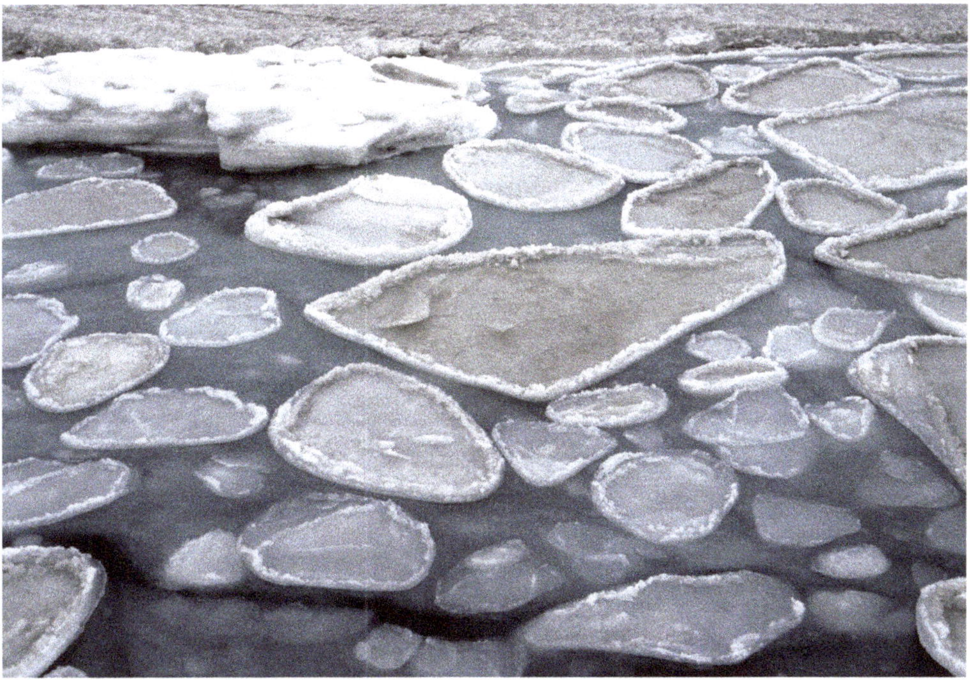

Fig. 1.10 — Pancake ice (Photo courtesy of Jim Mastro)

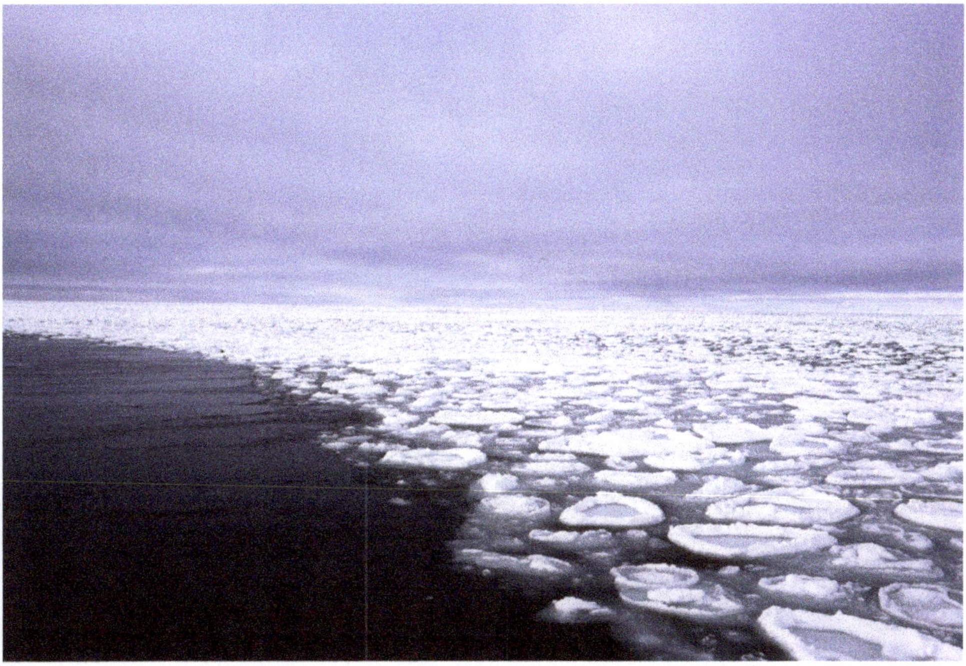

Fig. 1.11 — Sea ice sheets that break up and move with the wind and current are called pack ice. (Photo courtesy of Margaret Amsler)

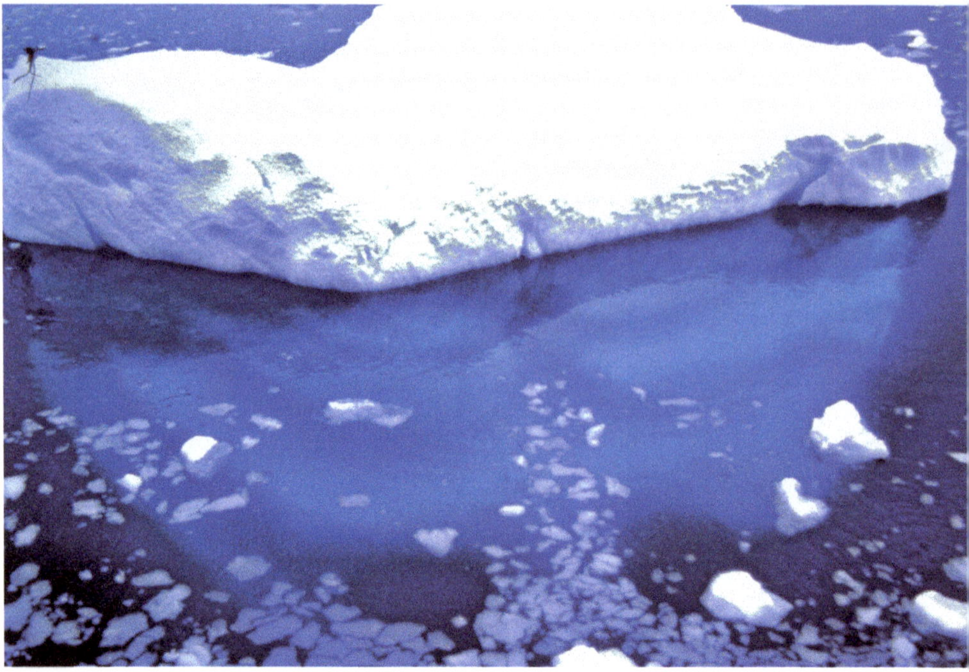

Fig. 1.12 — Larger ice floes can be dangerous for divers below.

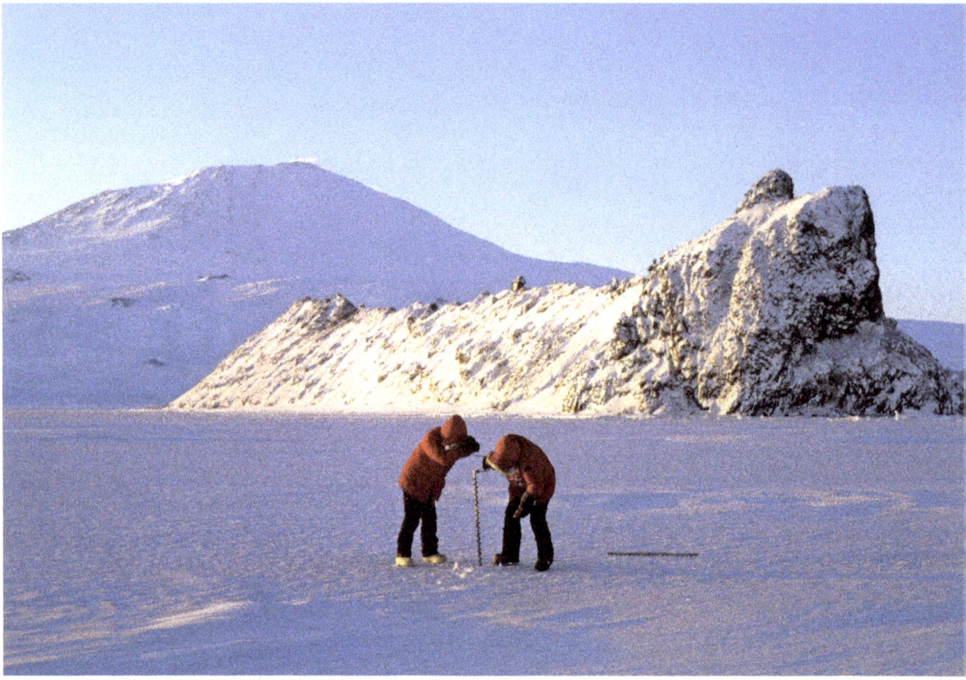

Fig. 1.13 — Fast ice is frozen to the shoreline. (Photo courtesy of Jim Mastro)

CHAPTER 2
Training

Ice diving can be a demanding and highly technical endeavor. It is difficult to state a set of prerequisites for entry into ice-diving training because it can vary widely between people, but certainly the diver must be very comfortable in the water. It is suggested that as a minimum the diver be certified as an advanced diver, have at least 25 logged open-water dives, and have prior drysuit training in open water.

Students in training should be expected to provide the usual open-water diving equipment, which additionally should include a drysuit, a scuba cylinder with a dual regulator valve (or a separate pony cylinder with regulator), two single-hose regulators appropriate for the water temperature, two dive lights, and a safety harness. The instructor may provide some of the equipment above in addition to downlines with flashers, safety lines, clips, ice-cutting equipment, ice screws, emergency equipment, and shelter. Recreational ice-diving training courses typically require a minimum of three open-water training dives.

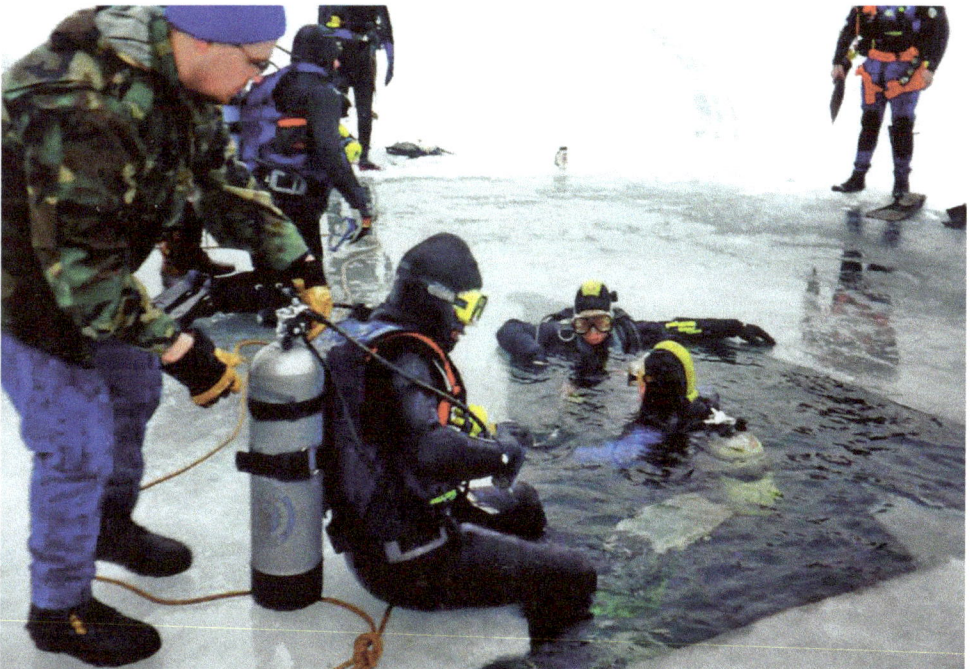

Fig. 2.1 — Formal ice-diving training is absolutely necessary for anyone wishing to dive under the ice. (Photo courtesy of Frank Morrow)

Classroom Curriculum

A sample outline of topics to be discussed in the classroom is provided. The length of classroom presentations will be dictated by the level of training required.

A. Cold Weather Environment
- Climate and weather temperature extremes
- Orientation to local conditions
- Wind chill
- Frostbite
- Hypothermia
- Sunburn, snow blindness

B. Cold Water Environment
- Physics of water
- Fresh- and saltwater ice formation
- Types of ice
- Seasonal stratification in lakes
- Orientation to local conditions

C. Equipment
- Thermal protection: drysuits and undergarments
- Accessories: hoods, gloves, mitts, mask, fins, knife
- Weight and buoyancy systems
- Cylinders and valves
- Regulators
- Lights, gauges, batteries
- Safety harness and tether lines, carabiners
- Tender equipment: layering for warmth and flexibility, boots, gloves
- Emergency equipment: first aid, oxygen, warm blankets, hot water, communications
- Hole-cutting equipment: chain saws, ice screws, shovels
- Shelter, heating

D. Ice-Diving Operations
- Evaluating ice conditions
- Preparing the dive site
- Cutting and clearing the dive hole
- Erecting a shelter

E. Dive Planning and Personnel
- Obtaining a weather forecast
- Tenders duties and responsibilities
- Safety diver responsibilities
- Dive plan review
- Line-pull signals
- Altitude diving considerations

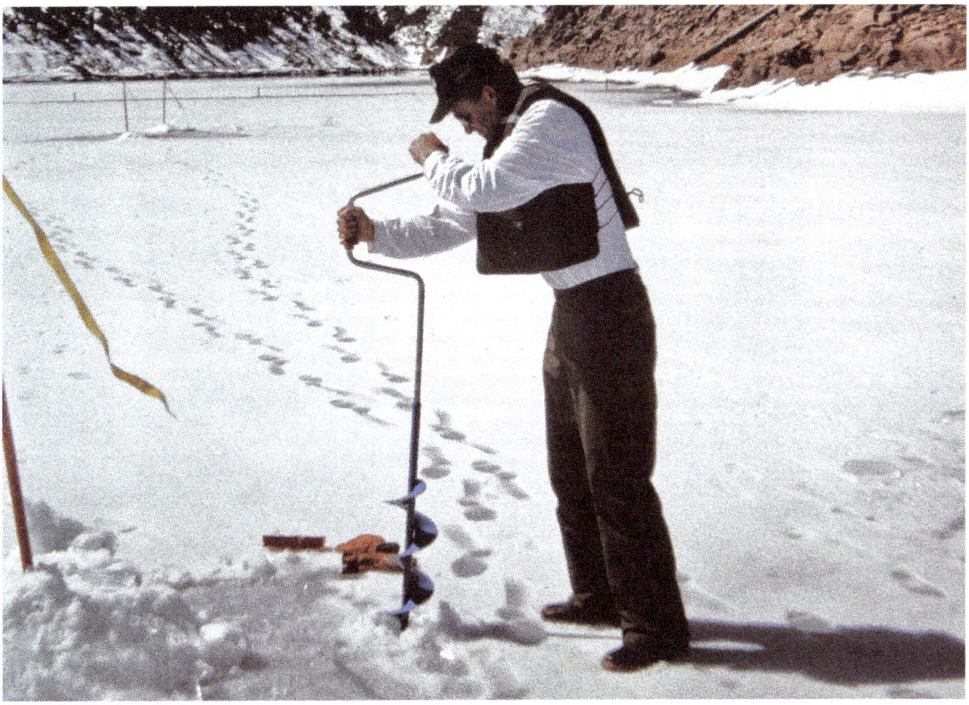

Fig. 2.2 — The ice-diving instructor will normally provide equipment such as a hole-drilling auger . . .

F. The Dive
- Suiting up
- Entry techniques
- Descent
- Buoyancy control
- Air management
- Communications with buddy and surface personnel
- Exit

G. Safety and Emergency Procedures
- Environmental hazards: currents, wind, visibility, cold
- Entanglement
- Regulator freeze up
- Inflator valve malfunction
- Dropped or lost weight belt
- Flooded drysuit
- Loss of dive hole

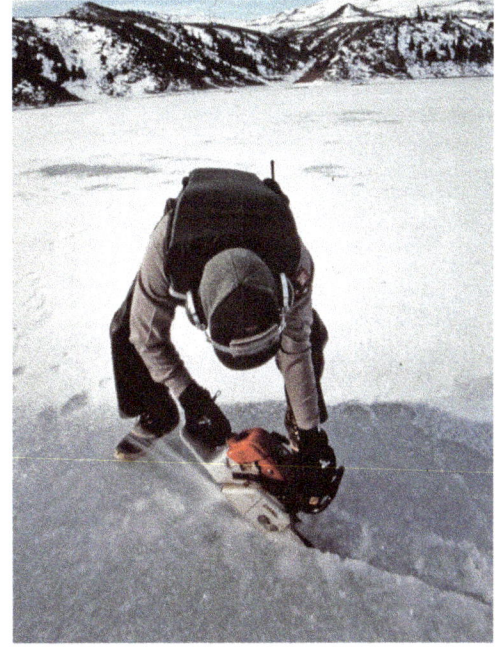

Fig. 2.3 — . . . and a chainsaw.

- Locating a lost diver, deploying the safety diver
- Diver rescue
- First aid, oxygen administration
- Emergency evacuation

Confined-Water Training

Confined-water (pool) training is considered to be optional by many ice-diving instructors. It is beneficial, however, if the instructor is not familiar with the students' skills in drysuit techniques, regulator recovery and switching, and buoyancy control.

If required, confined-water sessions should be conducted to familiarize participants with drysuit use, including problem solving, entries and exits, switching over from a freezing regulator, line-pull communications with the tender, and lost diver/lost exit hole procedures. Pool covers can be used to simulate the overhead environment provided by ice.

Drysuit Training

Drysuits are complex pieces of diving equipment and require training to become familiar and comfortable with their use. You should complete a thorough drysuit training course before attempting to use a drysuit. While drysuits are not particularly difficult to use, there are a number of special procedures you should learn from a qualified instructor. Divers accustomed to wearing wetsuits may find a drysuit to be uncomfortable and cumbersome at first for several reasons. First, drysuits generally consist of two layers — an outer waterproof suit that covers an inner layer of undergarments — so they can be somewhat bulky out of water. Second, for waterproofing, seals at the neck and wrists must fit snugly against the skin to keep the water out of the suit. You will become more used to these seals with time.

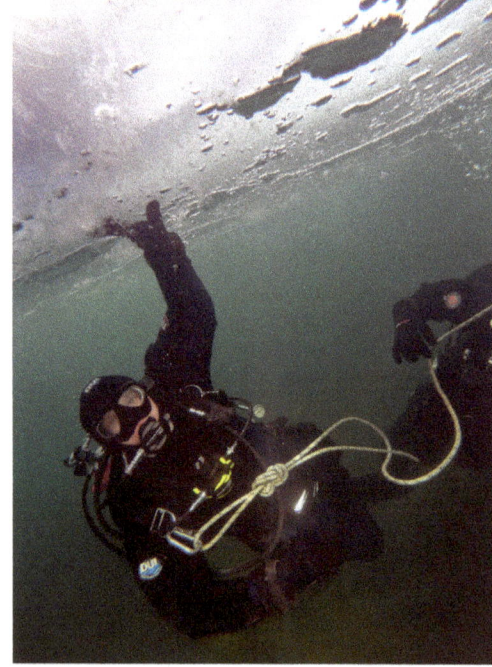

Fig. 2.4 – Drysuit training and skill development is part of the ice diver curriculum. (Photo courtesy of Frank Morrow)

Suggested Drysuit Skills

Divers should be able to demonstrate the following skills:

- Procedures for doffing and donning a drysuit
- Drysuit trim and buoyancy adjustment
- Drysuit diving descents and ascents without the use of a line
- Drysuit finning techniques
- Control of buoyancy throughout the dive and the ability to make a hovering stop at 15 fsw (5 msw)
- Proficiency in disconnecting/connecting drysuit and buoyancy compensator inflation valves underwater
- Ability to rapidly exhaust gas from drysuit
- Partial dropping of weights
- Procedures for dealing with inverted position from air in the feet, rapid ascent, and lost diver under ice
- Ability to remove dive gear at surface
- Postdive maintenance of drysuit, seals, and zipper lubrication

Ice Diving Open-Water Training

A minimum of three ice dives should be conducted in initial training. The first ice dive will be spent with a thorough orientation and preparation of the site. Dive holes must be cut, shelters erected, and emergency equipment staged. Trainees should rotate with surface tenders and personnel so that everyone gets a chance to act in all roles. The dive will consist

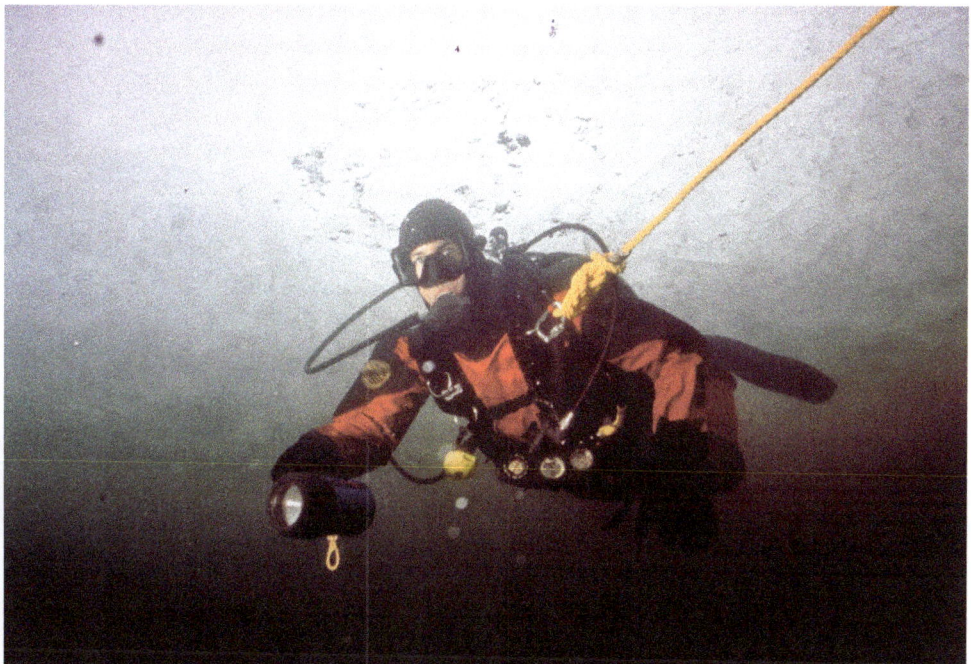

Fig. 2.5 — Open-water training includes close observation of divers by an instructor. (Photo courtesy of John Brooks)

of a limited (i.e., 50 ft./15 m) horizontal distance from the entry hole with a maximum of two trainees per instructor. This is essentially a familiarization dive so that the trainees understand the complexity and time involved with conducting an ice dive. Buoyancy skills, gas management, and line-pull signals with the tenders are to be practiced.

The subsequent dives will stress line signals, buoyancy control, navigation, problem solving, and emergency procedures drills. Specific scenarios can be constructed and acted out by the trainees under the supervision of the instructional staff. Careful practice of simulated suit blow-up, disconnecting low-pressure inflator hose, lost or

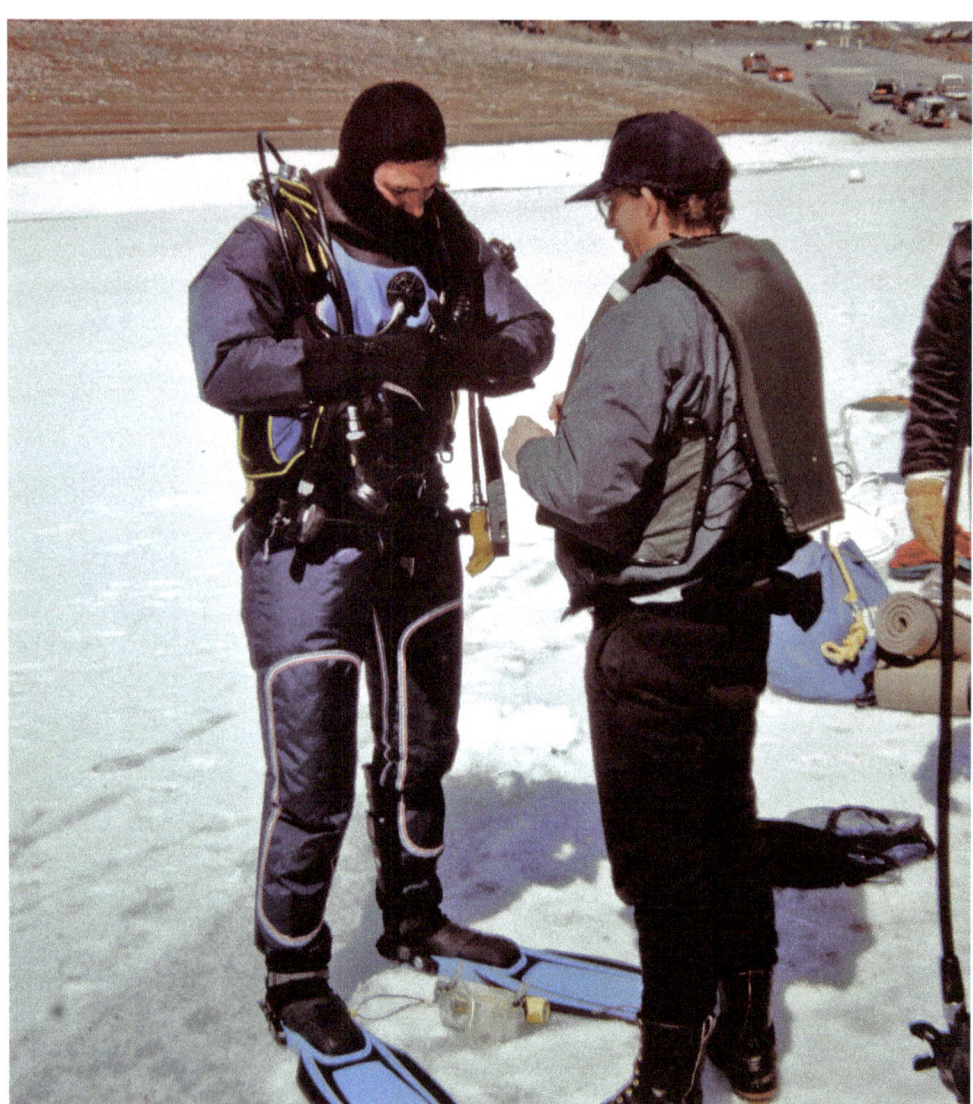

Fig. 2.6 — A tender and diver review the dive plan and safety checks.

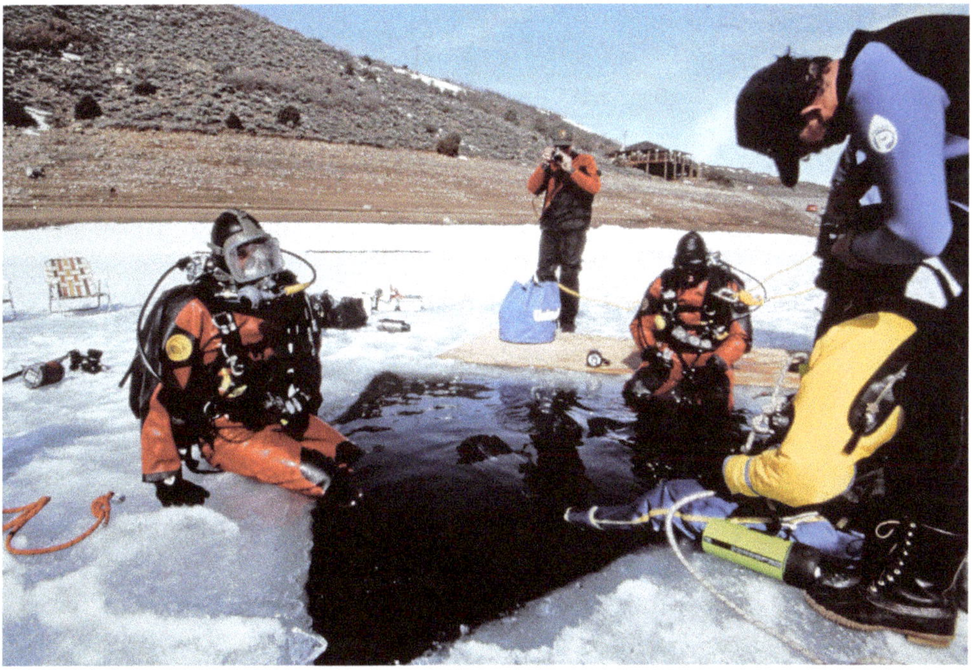

Fig. 2.7 — Advanced ice-diving training might include the use of a full-face mask . . .

dropped weight belt, simulated lost diver procedures, simulated regulator malfunction and swap to secondary regulator, and rescues can be conducted. The postdive debriefing is a key part of all dive training.

All participants should rotate through the various support and diver positions so they have some training and appreciation for the responsibilities involved. Students should not be allowed to actually be responsible for tending but can assist under supervision. The instructor will, of course, be in a position to supervise and evaluate the ice-diving training. This might include both surface and underwater supervision, so the presence of appropriately trained assistants is essential.

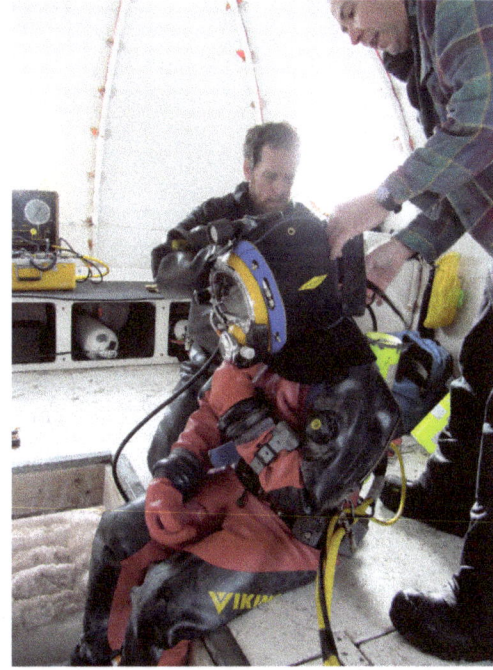

Fig. 2.8 — . . . or even surface-supplied diving gear.

CHAPTER 3
Equipment for Ice Diving

Diving is an equipment-intensive activity. Ice diving requires an extensive amount of additional equipment because of the cold weather and water, the remote locations involved, and the presence of an overhead obstruction during the dive. It is important for ice divers to understand the requirements and options for equipment to make informed purchases and decisions.

Thermal Protection for Divers

Diving is not fun if you are cold. It also can be hazardous if a diver gets hypothermia. Divers in cold water have a higher air-consumption rate, expend more energy, and can become more fatigued than divers in warmer water. Cold water also decreases a diver's ability to perform complex tasks that require manual dexterity. Drysuits offer benefits such as increasing the warmth and comfort of the diver, helping conserve energy, which results in less fatigue, and keeping divers warmer on the surface between dives than a wetsuit does, especially in the wind.

Neoprene wetsuits can be worn on shorter, shallow ice dives, but modern drysuits are preferable. A neoprene wetsuit compresses dramatically with depth due to the air spaces in the material, which significantly reduces the insulating properties of the material. Most drysuit materials do not compress with depth, and air is added to the inside of the suit to overcome the compression of the air spaces in the undergarments. This means that the insulative value of the drysuit does not change greatly with depth as it does with a wetsuit.

Drysuits require more care and maintenance than wetsuits, most of which you can do yourself. They also require training in their proper use and care.

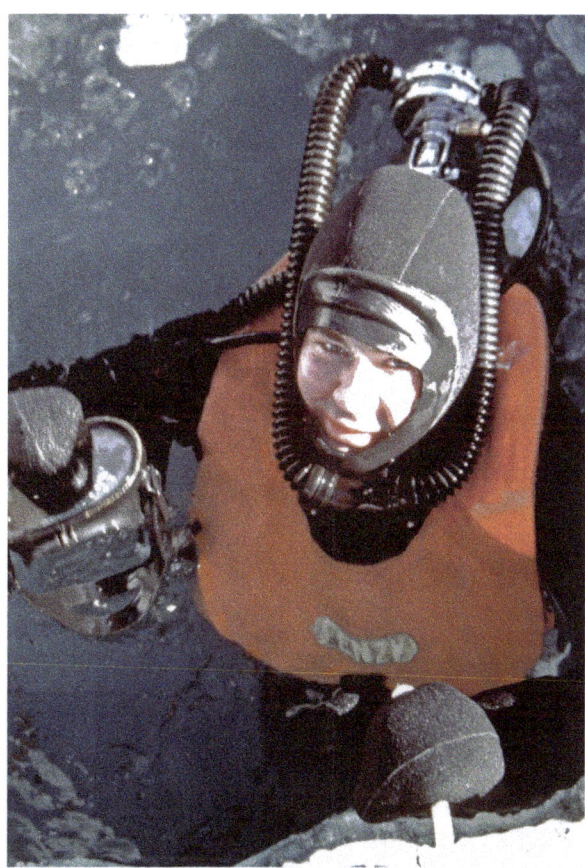

Fig. 3.1 — Before the advent of drysuits, wetsuits were worn under the ice. (Photo © Dale T. Andersen, all rights reserved)

Types of Drysuits

Drysuits are made out of several different types of materials, each having its advantages and disadvantages. The original type of drysuit material is closed-cell (or foam) neoprene, the same material used to make wetsuits. The benefits of this material are that it has good stretch, provides considerable insulation without undergarments, and is relatively inexpensive. The disadvantages include the considerable buoyancy of the material, which requires a large amount of additional weight, and the fact that this material compresses with depth, which reduces its insulation effects and creates large changes in buoyancy.

Closed-cell neoprene drysuits are constructed similar to wetsuits, using glue and stitching. The seams will deteriorate with age but are relatively easy to repair. The material is also subject to punctures from barnacles, sea urchin spines, and other sharp objects. However, the neoprene is usually covered with nylon to promote resistance to wear by abrasion. The neck and wrist seals are usually made of neoprene as well, but latex seals can be specially ordered.

Crushed neoprene drysuits use thick neoprene that has been compressed. The advantage to this material is that it is thinner and denser, which decreases its inherent buoyancy yet makes it stronger while retaining its stretch. This type of suit fits close to the body, which decreases the drag associated with baggy suits. The seams may be glued, stitched, and/or taped. The seals can be constructed of either neoprene, latex, or silicone. These suits are expensive but will provide many years of service. An example of this type of drysuit is the DUI CF200.

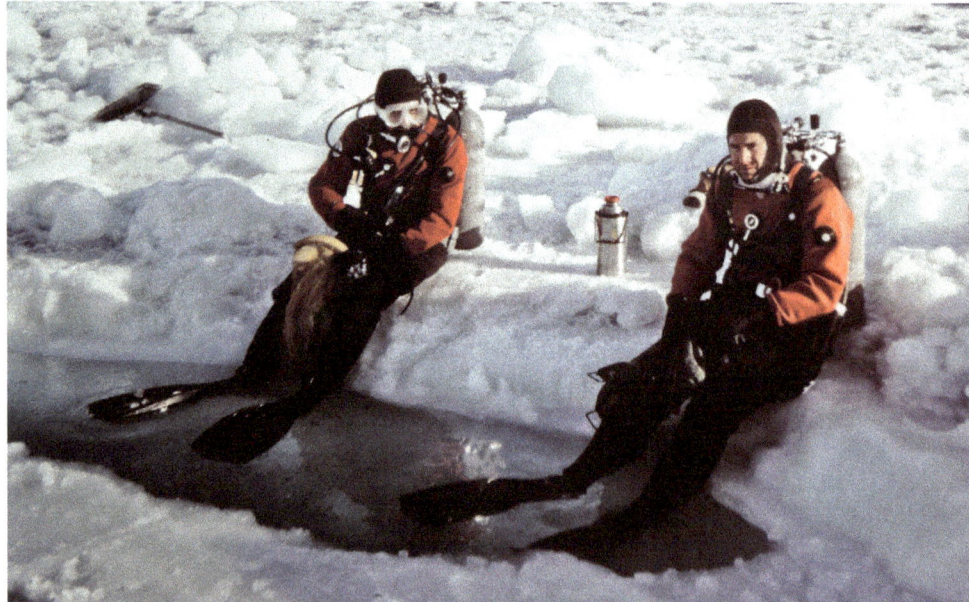

Fig. 3.2 — The DUI CF200 is a crushed neoprene drysuit.

The remaining types of drysuits fall into the category of shell suits. These drysuits provide no buoyancy and minimal, if any, insulation, serving only to keep the diver dry. Insulation is achieved by wearing undergarments beneath the drysuit.

The first type of shell suit is made of trilaminate material, which is composed of three layers: nylon, polyester, and Cordura on the outside. The material is very strong, resistant to abrasion, and lightweight, but it does not stretch much. It rolls into a very small package and dries very quickly, which makes it desirable for travel. Trilaminate drysuits usually have latex wrist and neck seals. Popular examples are the DUI TLS350 and the Santi E.Lite and E.Motion suits.

Urethane-backed nylon is a more economical material sometimes used in shell suits. It has properties similar to the trilaminate material but is thinner and stiffer. The material does not stretch, so these suits often appear somewhat baggy since they must fit more loosely to allow entry and exit from the suit.

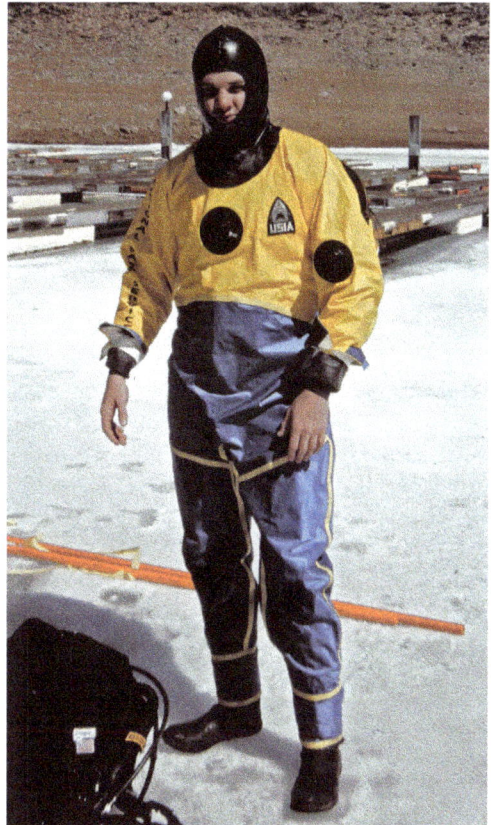

Fig. 3.3 — A variety of shell suits are available that keep the diver dry, such as this one with a back zipper.

The final type of shell drysuit material is rubber, which is usually made from a combination of natural and synthetic rubber, with a polyester lining. The material is bonded together under heat and pressure or by a chemical vulcanization process, which produces a very strong bond. These suits have some stretch, which makes them easy to don and comfortable to wear. The material is strong, easy to patch, dries very quickly, and lasts many years. The user usually can make repairs to the suit at the dive site. Various thicknesses are available for the range of diving needs. A popular example of a vulcanized rubber drysuit is the Viking brand.

Features of Drysuits

All drysuits share some essential features such as a waterproof zipper, inflation and exhaust valves, and neck and wrist seals, but many options and styles are available.

The waterproof zipper is the most critical — and expensive — part of a drysuit. It should be large and strong. The longer the zipper the more expensive it is. The length

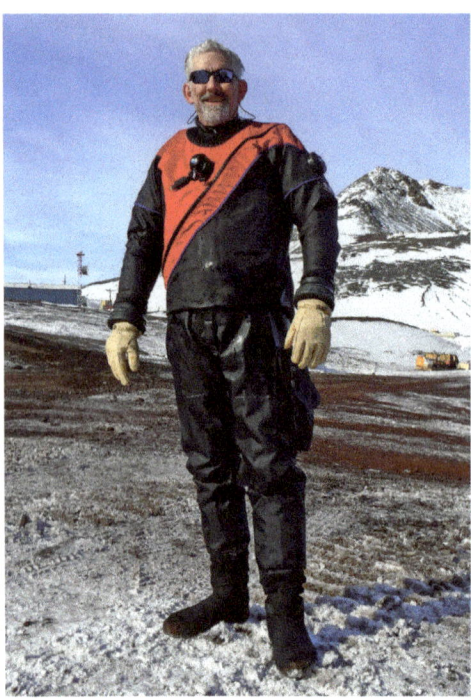 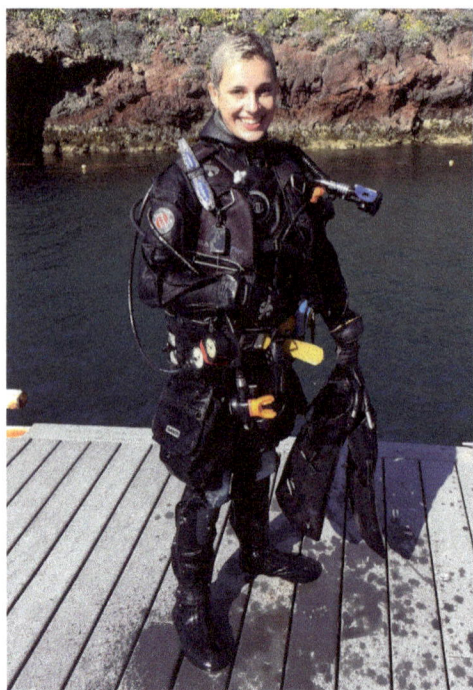

Fig. 3.4 – The DUI TLS350 trilaminate suit (left) has a self-donning front entry that allows the user to doff and don the suit themselves. (Photo courtesy of Steve Rupp) The Santi E-series drysuits (right) are made from a variety of fabrics that are lightweight but durable.

of the zipper is primarily a function of where it is placed on the suit. Drysuit zippers can be placed horizontally across the front or back of the shoulders, diagonally from one shoulder across the chest to the opposite hip, or from the back under the crotch to the front.

The most common location of the zipper is along the back between the shoulders. This requires the assistance of your buddy to open and close the zipper when dressing in and out. This zipper location can restrict movement if it is not long enough, and the zipper can take some physical abuse from the buoyancy compensator rubbing against it.

The self-donning type of drysuit has a zipper that runs diagonally across the

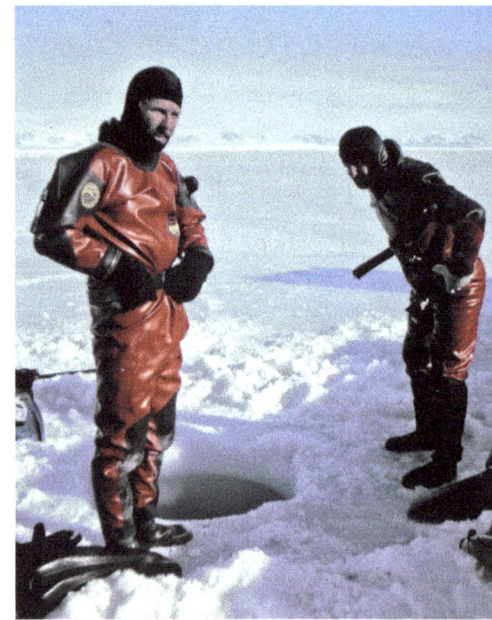

Fig. 3.5 — Viking makes a durable vulcanized rubber drysuit.

chest. The advantages to this are that the diver can completely dress in and out of the suit without assistance and can easily open it between dives. Divers must take care while diving to not lay on the bottom and get sediment into the zipper. Some suits have a zipper guard, which is a layer of extra material that protects the waterproof zipper.

Drysuit neck and wrist seals are made of either neoprene or latex or silicone rubber. Neoprene neck seals are usually 1/8 inch (3 mm) thick, and the wrist seals can vary from 1/8 to 1/4 inch (3-7 mm) thick. The smooth side of the neoprene seals against the diver's skin. They can be configured to either lie flat against the skin (cone shaped) or be rolled under an inch or so to seal against the skin. Neoprene should not be trimmed to make the seals larger but should be stretched slowly and gradually. Neoprene seals are difficult to repair in the field because the material must be totally dry before repairs can be made, and the cement requires time to cure. See the manufacturer's recommendations before repairing or altering your seals.

Latex rubber seals are made of natural rubber, are thin, stretchy, and strong, and come in a variety of thicknesses. They have very good resistance to tears and abrasions but are not very resistant to oils or aging due to exposure to sunlight. These seals can be trimmed to fit using sharp scissors, but if you are not experienced with this procedure, it is best to let a dealer do it. Silicone seals have the advantage of being very stretchable and resistant to ultraviolet light and ozone but are not as resistant as latex seals to tearing or punctures.

New drysuit divers often will mistake a correct-fitting neck seal as too tight and may trim it back too far. It should fit snug but not so tight as to restrict breathing and

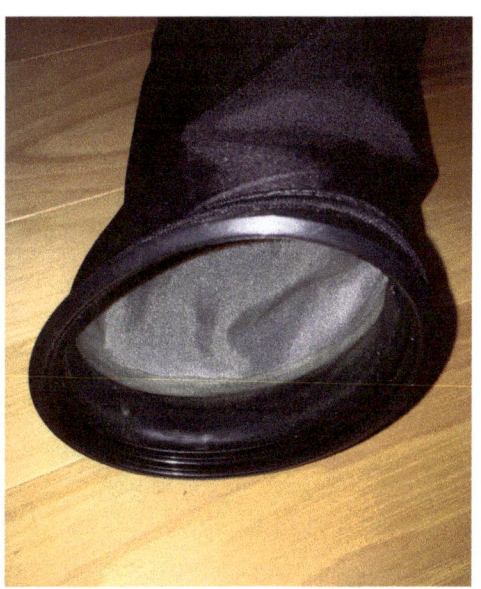 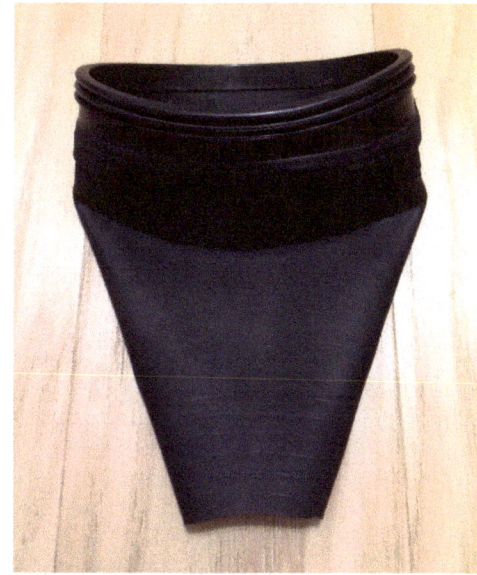

Fig. 3.6 — DUI's ZipSeals system allows the user to change a damaged wrist or neck seal easily in the field. Pictured are a) drysuit sleeve with ZipSeal grooves, b) latex ZipSeal showing rings for trimming to size.

circulation. If you are in doubt, see your dealer. Latex seals are vulnerable to puncture from sharp fingernails, jewelry, and marine life. However, they are not difficult to repair in the field.

All drysuit seals are subject to wear and tear and will need to be replaced periodically. You should replace them when they start to leak or if they become torn.

Drysuit inflation and deflation valves allow the diver to control the volume of air in the drysuit, which affects both the buoyancy and thermal protection of the diver. The inflator valve operates similarly to a BC low-pressure inflator mechanism. It is usually mounted in the chest region of the suit. A quick-disconnect low-pressure hose from the regulator first stage attaches to the inflator valve for power inflation. Some inflator valves will rotate to allow the low-pressure hose to come over or under the arm on either side of the body.

Inflator valves can freeze up and cause free flow if moisture is in the mechanism. Valves should be dry, and any snow or water should be blown dry off an inflator hose before attachment. Divers should use only brief (i.e., one second) bursts of air from the valve and avoid depressing it for longer periods. Holding the valve open for extended periods can cause free flow. Divers should practice disconnecting the inflator hose in case it freezes up.

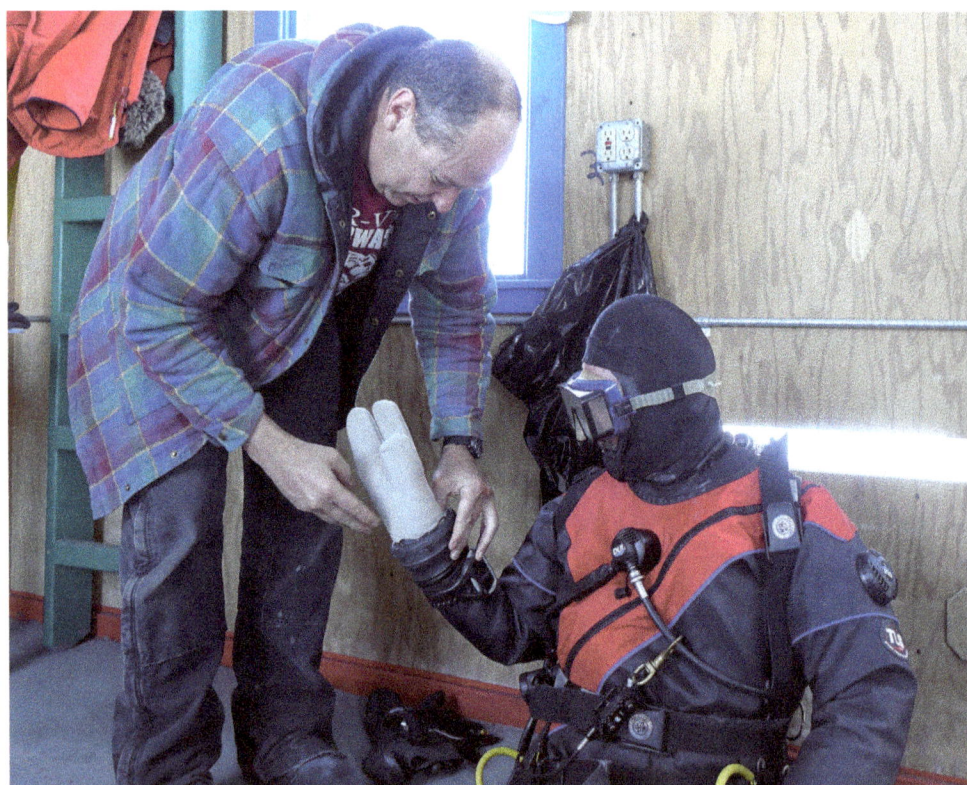

Fig. 3.7 — Inflator and exhaust valves on a drysuit

The exhaust valve is usually located on the upper-arm area of the drysuit. A manual exhaust valve must be operated by hand, which requires pressing on it to release air on ascent. The diver can adjust automatic exhaust valves to control the rate of exhaust from the drysuit. By setting it in the open position before ascent, the valve will automatically vent off the expanding air as the ambient pressure decreases. The valve must be at the highest point of the drysuit to allow all of the air to escape. Most automatic valves have a manual override feature, which allows the valve to be fully opened by depressing the valve by hand.

Custom sizing is available for most drysuits but usually is not necessary. The size you will use is based on your height, weight, and shoe size. There should be enough room for the dive undergarments and to allow bending and squatting without discomfort.

Accessories

Most drysuits have attached boots made of heavy-duty neoprene or molded sole rubber. Most attached boots are quite large and require the use of fins with large foot pockets. Some models have thinner attached "socks" that are meant to be used with separate heavy-duty boots. Knee pads are desirable, as this is often a location subject to considerable wear. Pockets also can be ordered in various sizes and locations on the drysuit.

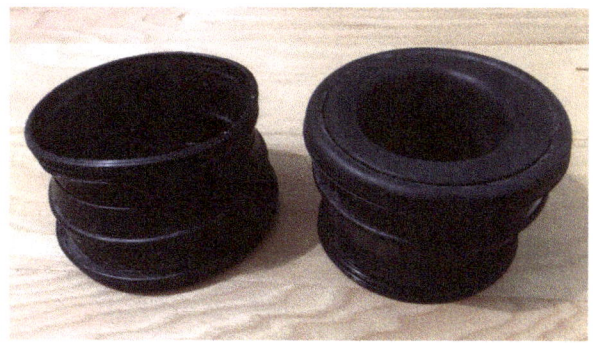

Fig. 3.8 — Heavy-duty rubber rings can be fitted to latex seals to allow for attachment of a variety of gloves or mitts.

A hood is required if the water is cold enough to warrant wearing a drysuit. Standard neoprene wetsuit hoods can be used with some drysuits. A more preferred hood is one made especially to seal against the neck seal of the drysuit. These hoods usually have a short neck and use skin-in neoprene around the neck and sometimes around the face to provide a good seal against

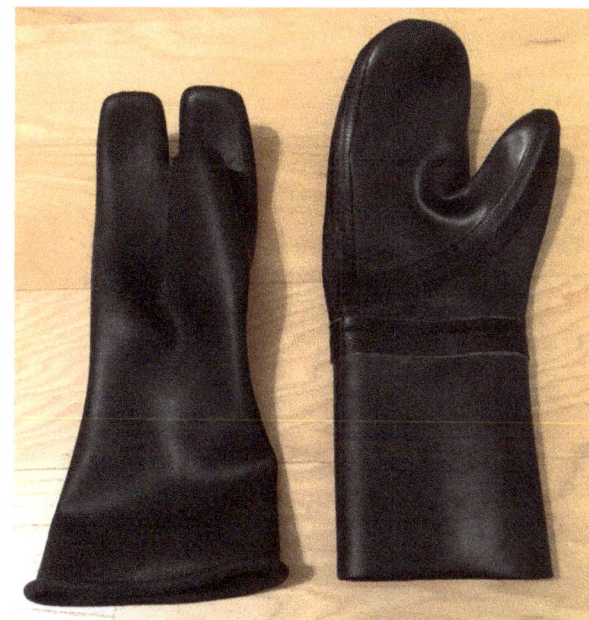

Fig. 3.9 — Latex (left) and rubber (right) mitts can be stretched over the rubber rings to provide a dry seal.

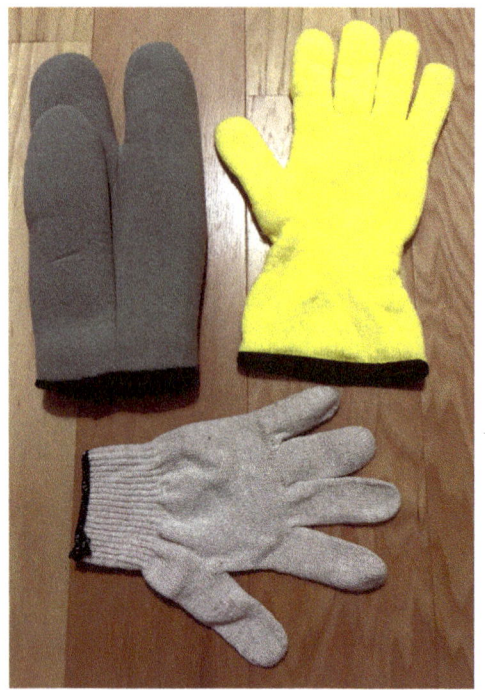
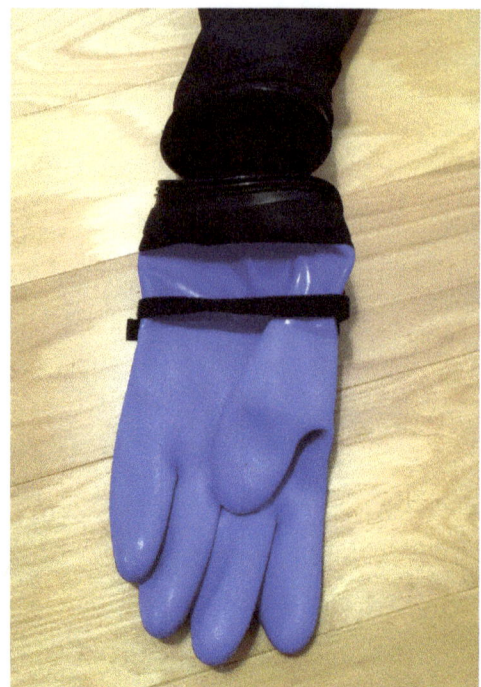

Fig. 3.10 — A variety of layered undergloves provides maximum warmth but limits dexterity.

Fig. 3.11 — DUI ZipGlove system

water intrusion. Other hoods incorporate a longer neck skirt for tucking into collars built into the drysuit.

There are also dry hoods made out of neoprene or latex that can be attached directly to the drysuit. The latex hood can be used with an insulated liner or over another neoprene hood and works well in extremely cold environments. They generally do not seal against beards or on people with very thin faces.

Regular neoprene gloves or mitts may be used with a drysuit. Colder water dictates the use of thicker gloves. Gauntlet-style gloves are a good choice to give protection around latex wrist seals. Three-fingered mitts are warmer than five-fingered gloves because the surface area that can be cooled is reduced. However, dexterity is reduced with mitts as compared with gloves.

In very cold ice-diving conditions, special dry gloves are available that seal against rings on the arm of the drysuit. Liners worn under the dry gloves provide insulation to the hands for warmth. To prevent glove squeeze and to promote warmth, short pieces of surgical tubing or cocktail straws can be inserted under the wrist seals to provide a conduit for air to exchange from the suit to the gloves. In some cases the wrist seals can be trimmed back to allow for more exchange of air, but if the glove leaks, this will allow water to enter the drysuit.

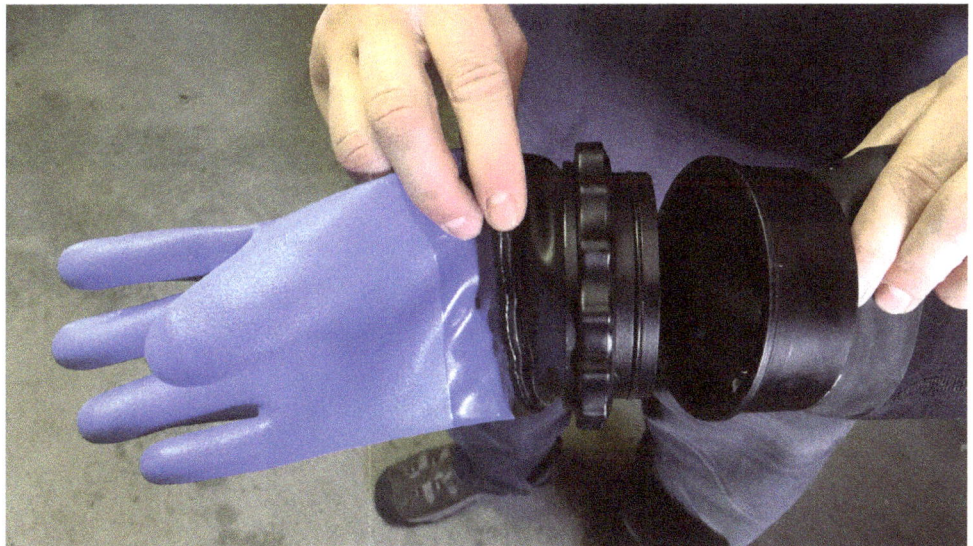

Fig. 3.12 — The SI Tech Glove Lock system is easy to don with a twist and lock mechanism.

Some dry glove systems require a tender to stretch the glove and place it over the wrist ring on the drysuit (see Fig. 3.7). Others allow for easy self-donning and removal by the diver. The SI Tech Glove Lock system is easy to don with a twist and lock mechanism. DUI's ZipGloves system mounts to the wrist of the drysuit before the user dons the suit and can be a little difficult for dexterity while donning the rest of the equipment if thick liners are worn underneath.

Undergarments

Drysuits are designed to keep you dry, while undergarments help keep you warm. Some thicker neoprene drysuits (1/4 inch or 7 mm) are worn without undergarments, but all shell suits require that some type of insulation be worn underneath. Many types of undergarments are available, made of various material types with different features and prices.

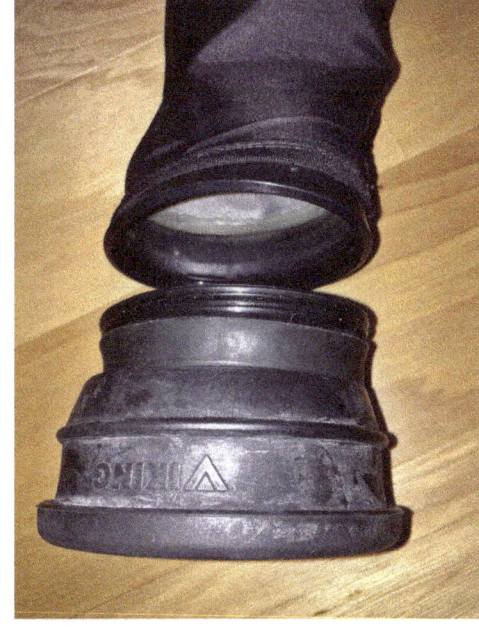

Fig. 3.13 — The Viking rubber rings can be attached to a DUI ZipSeal to allow for the use of large mitts.

The function of undergarments is to trap air against your body to be warmed. The colder the water, the thicker or more layers of undergarments are required. Many drysuit divers wear a thin set of polypropylene or bamboo fiber liners under their thicker undergarments. This type of material helps to wick away any moisture from the body. It is also much easier to launder the thin liners than the bulkier undergarments.

Most drysuit undergarments are available in a variety of thicknesses that can be chosen depending upon the temperature of the water, the physiology of the diver, and the anticipated level of activity. Undergarments add bulk, and they must fit comfortably under the drysuit without being too tight. The one-piece jumpsuit style is the most common and comfortable configuration of dive wear. Two-piece undergarments allow for more flexibility in layering. Many brands have thumb loops at the wrist and ankle stirrups that the diver places over

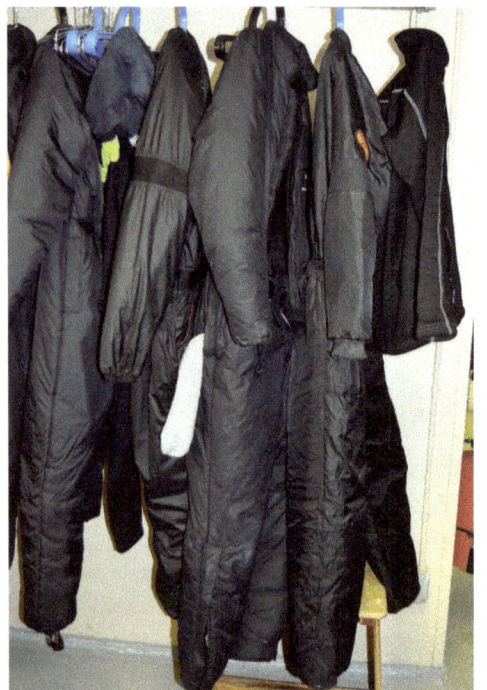

Fig. 3.14 — Thick undergarments and boots are worn under a drysuit when ice diving.

the thumbs or heels when donning the drysuit. This keeps the sleeves and legs of the undergarments from being pulled up the arm or leg when pulling on the drysuit. The thumb loops must be tucked under the wrist seal to keep from leaking.

The first type of undergarment is called fleece, which is also known as woolly bears or synthetic pile (i.e., Polartec). This type of material is somewhat bulky and provides good insulation on the surface. However, it compresses with depth, which decreases its

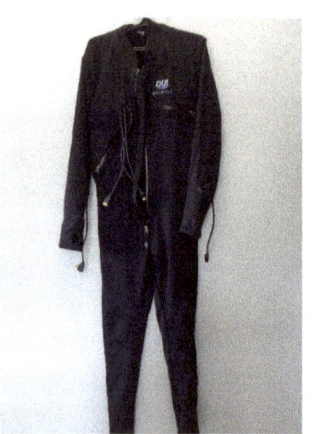 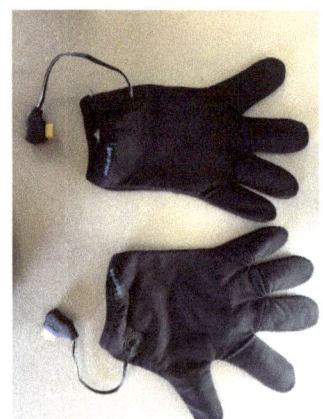 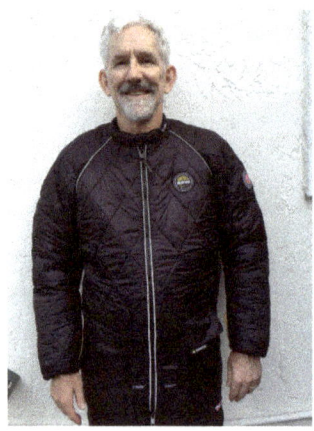

Fig. 3.15 — From left: DUI BlueHeat electric jumpsuit and gloves and Santi heated undersuit

insulative value. It also loses its insulation when wet. Lint from this material can clog the exhaust valve of the drysuit and cause it to leak.

The second type of undergarment is open-cell foam. It offers slightly greater insulation than fleece, does not compress greatly with depth, does not produce lint, and is easy to launder. It functions when slightly damp but will not insulate when wet. Some undergarments are made out of a wool blend.

Another type of material used in drysuit undergarments is called radiant barrier or radiant insulating material. This type of material uses an aluminum polyethylene film type of fabric, like a "space blanket," which reflects heat back to your body. It is sandwiched between nylon on the outside and soft polyester on the inside. It functions well when wet and is easy to clean.

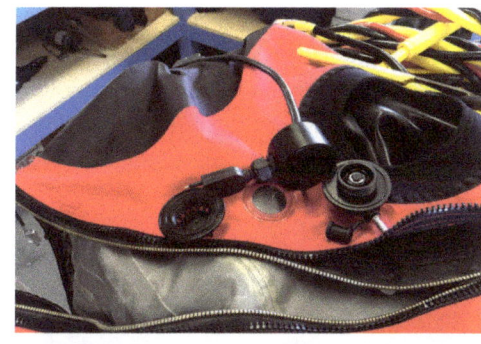
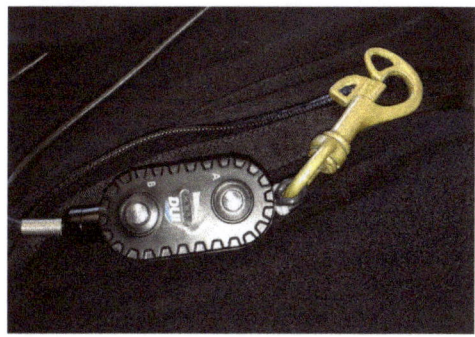

Fig. 3.16 — Electric heated undergarments require a port that is installed under the inflation valve (top) and is operated by a controller (bottom) that allows for multiple power settings.

The final type of undergarment is made of Thinsulate, which is usually coated with nylon on the outside and soft cotton or polyester on the inside. It is a very good insulator, even when wet. It is relatively thin, breathable, and very comfortable. It is also fairly expensive. Thinsulate must be laundered carefully, according to the manufacturer's instructions. Some divers wear a thin wetsuit under the drysuit and report that it keeps them sufficiently warm. Various types of socks and boots are available as well.

Electric heated undergarment systems are now available to wear under drysuits. The DUI BlueHeat system consists of a jumpsuit liner with heating pads, a smart battery system and controller, and heated gloves and socks. The battery pack is

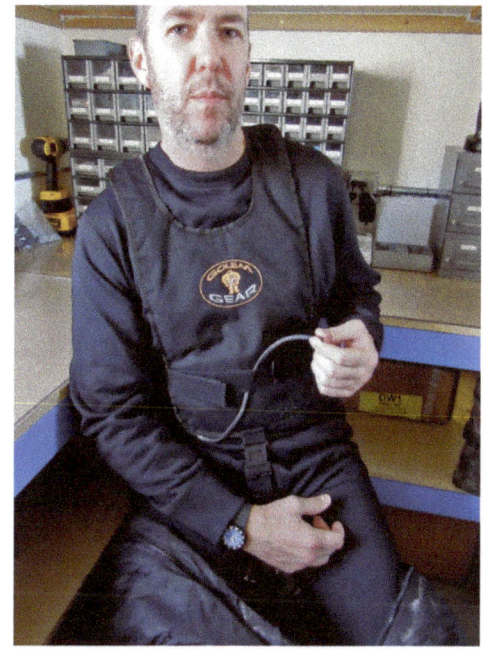

Fig. 3.17 — A Golem Gear heated undervest

large and somewhat heavy and is strapped to the diver's cylinder. Thermalution makes a simple, electric, battery-powered undersuit that incorporates the batteries inside the drysuit. Santi has heated undersuits, vests, and gloves, which are powered by external batteries of various capacities depending upon the conditions. Golem Gear makes a heated vest and glove inserts that are powered by lithium batteries.

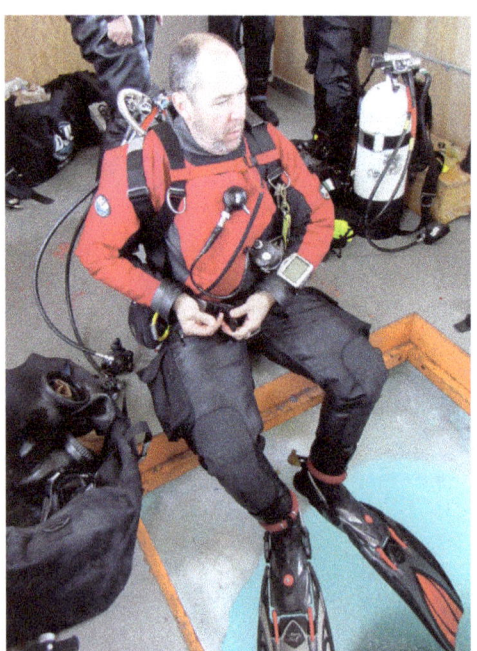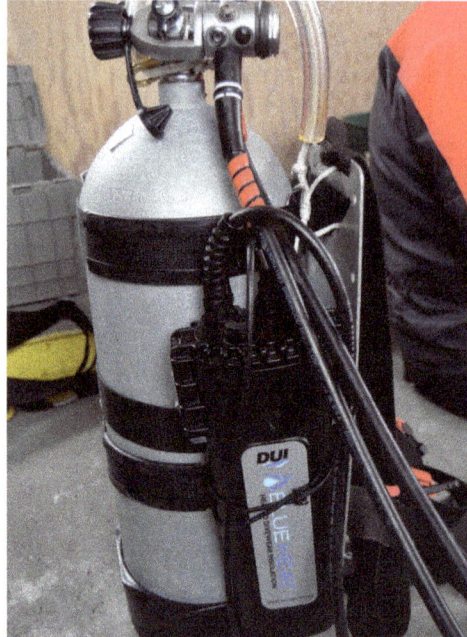

Fig. 3.18 — The external battery canister can be worn similar to a sidemount cylinder (left) or attached to the main scuba cylinder (right).

Weight and Buoyancy Systems

Drysuits require a considerable amount of weight to be worn to achieve neutral buoyancy. However, a common misconception about diving dry is the need to add tremendous amounts of weight to the belt. Depending upon the diver's physical characteristics, the type of drysuit, the type of cylinder used, and the type and thickness of undergarments, many divers add only a small amount of weight to achieve neutral buoyancy.

The proper way to use a drysuit is with the minimal amount of air inside the suit necessary to avoid a squeeze. Divers who put excessive amounts of air in the drysuit require more weight than would otherwise be needed, which can lead to buoyancy problems during the dive.

Standard weight belts, with lead weights of various sizes, will work with a drysuit. Depending upon the drysuit and undergarments, these type of weights may dig into the drysuit and the diver's hips and create discomfort. Soft weight belts that are filled with lead shot mold to the diver's body and are more comfortable. They are also easier on the drysuit material. Many buoyancy compensators also incorporate the ability to carry weights in releasable pockets.

To achieve proper buoyancy and trim characteristics, many divers redistribute some of their weight onto different parts of the body. One way to accomplish this is by the use of ankle weights. These one- to two-pound lead shot soft weights clip to each ankle and help to keep the feet from rising higher than the diver's head.

Another method of moving the weight around is by use of a weight and trim system. This weight belt incorporates shoulder straps that transfer the weight onto the diver's shoulders, which helps to relieve lower-back strain. The harness allows adjustment of the weights forward, backward, up, and down to keep the center of gravity below the center of buoyancy. Weights can be dropped or removed by using two quick-release mechanisms.

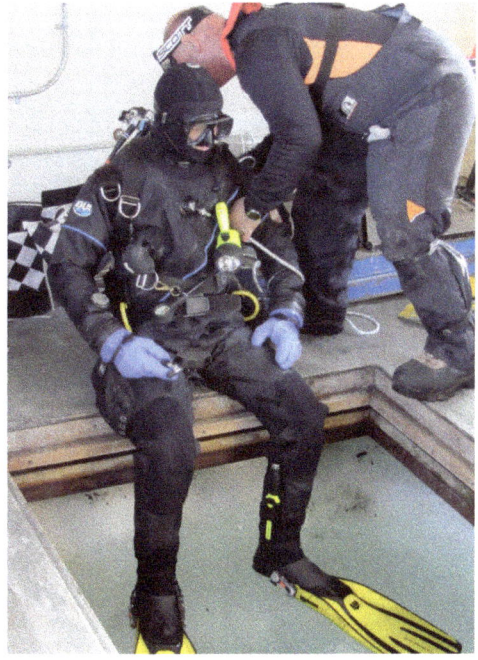

Fig. 3.19 — The DUI weight trim system has two separate weight-release handles (yellow) and supports the weight on the diver's shoulders.

The other part of any weight system is the buoyancy compensator (BC). A buoyancy compensator should always be used with a drysuit to facilitate surface swimming in open water and to be used in case the drysuit cannot hold air, the inflator valve malfunctions, or the drysuit totally floods with water. Many drysuit divers prefer a back-type BC, as it does not cover up or interfere with the drysuit valves. Exercise special care when using a power inflator in freezing water. Use only short bursts to avoid freeze up and free flow.

Care and Maintenance

Proper care and maintenance of your drysuit will prolong its useful life and provide many years of warm, comfortable diving. One of the most important steps is to thoroughly rinse the suit and its parts in freshwater after diving. If possible, have your buddy rinse you down with a garden hose while you are still in the suit. This keeps water from getting inside.

Use caution when removing a drysuit in freezing weather, as the zipper can become stiff and brittle. Open the zipper carefully and entirely. To remove a latex neck seal, reach through the top of the seal with both hands and spread open the neck seal. Lift the seal up and over the head. Be careful not to let fingernails dig into the seal. For a neoprene neck seal, first unroll the seal, then use the same method. To remove wrist seals, you can pull your hand out by turning the sleeve inside out, or you or your buddy can spread open the seal while you pull your hand through.

After you have removed the drysuit, close the zipper and hold the wrist seals together with the neck seal in a position above the rest of the suit. This way water will not get inside the suit while rinsing. Rinse the valves and zipper thoroughly. Blow dry the valves with compressed air after rinsing. If your suit got wet inside during the dive, rinse it as well.

Wash latex seals occasionally with a dilute solution of soapy water to remove body oils. It is best to hang the suit upside down in a shady area to dry, with the zipper open. Never hang your suit in the sun to dry, as this can damage the material. If the inside of the suit is wet, turn it inside out all the way to the boots and allow the inside to dry. Feel down into the boots to make sure they are dry. When the suit is dry, apply talcum powder to the latex seals to keep them from sticking.

The zipper is an important and expensive part of a drysuit. It requires proper care and maintenance to perform properly and last many years. Lubricating with wax has already been discussed. Anytime the zipper teeth become dirty, clean them with a toothbrush and soapy water before opening or closing the zipper. Use care when closing the zipper, as undergarments may get caught in the zipper and can cause damage to the teeth. If zipper teeth become out of alignment or broken, have a dealer check them prior to use. Check with the manufacturer for storage suggestions. Generally, store the suit with the zipper open.

Drysuits should be clean and dry before storage. The zipper should be open to avoid excessive compression on the sealing surfaces. Some manufacturers supply a protective cap to place over the inflator valve to keep the stem from puncturing the suit. Most suits should be rolled up and placed in a bag for storage. The drysuit manufacturer usually supplies the storage bags.

Service and Repairs

Eventually your suit will require service and repairs. The drysuit valves should be inspected and serviced according to manufacturer's instructions, which are usually every year. The valves should be disassembled and repaired only by factory-trained technicians.

The user can often perform simple repairs such as small punctures. Most manufacturers supply repair kits that contain glues and materials to match the type of drysuit that needs repair.

Replacement of seals can be more difficult and is best left to a qualified technician.

Manufacturers can perform leak tests to determine the source of water leaks in the drysuit.

To locate puncture holes yourself, you can close off the seals with bottles or cans and rubber bands, close the zipper, and fully inflate the suit. Larger holes or split seams can often be identified by listening carefully for escaping air. You can also brush on a dilute solution of soapy water and look for bubbles to form. Another method is to hold up sections of the drysuit to a bright light and look for holes. Mark punctures with a crayon or grease pencil.

Minor field patches can be applied on the inside of nylon fabric materials. Vulcanized rubber suits can often be permanently patched in as little as 10 minutes. Aquaseal can often be used to repair punctures and seams.

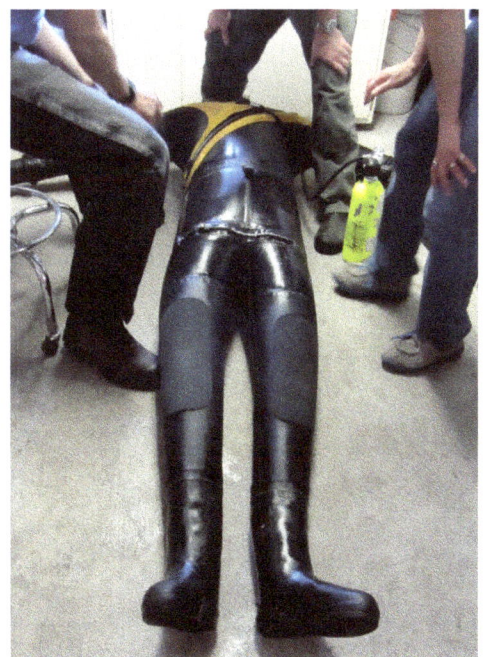

Fig. 3.20 — An inflated drysuit is checked for leaks using a soapy solution.

Cylinders and Valve Configurations

Ice diving requires a sufficient supply of gas to complete the intended dive plus a reserve amount of gas for potential emergencies. The minimum volume for the primary cylinder should be an 80- to 100-cubic-foot cylinder. It should be equipped with a Y- or H-valve configuration to allow for mounting two independent regulators on a single cylinder.

Modular valve systems can be expanded to change configurations as the diver requires. A basic K valve can be adapted to convert to an H valve, allowing for the attachment of primary and backup regulators. Either regulator can be independently isolated if there is a

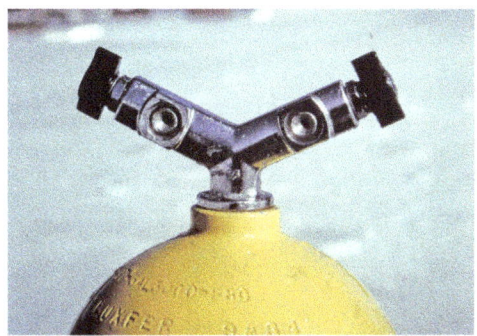

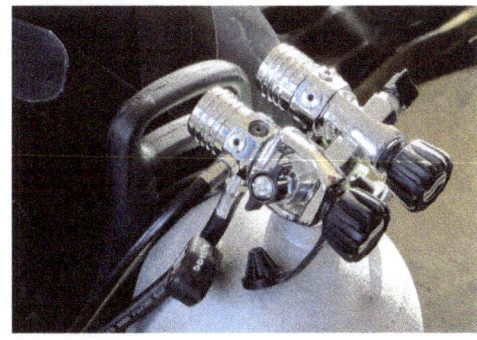

Fig. 3.21 — A Y valve (top) allows for the attachment of the separate regulators to a single cylinder (bottom).

malfunction. Double cylinder configurations can also be incorporated with these valve systems.

A secondary scuba cylinder or pony bottle — a small, approximately 15-cubic-foot cylinder — can be used with its own separate regulator in place of the valve configuration described above.

O-rings can become brittle in freezing conditions. Clean and lubricate them often, and inspect them for cracks.

Regulators

Double-hose regulators were utilized in many of the early ice dives but are not used today. They work well in freezing water but are not manufactured any longer, and parts are difficult to find for the older models. Many modern single-hose scuba regulators will not function well in cold or freezing water. Both the first and second stages can freeze. First-stage freezing can occur due to the expansion that occurs when air leaves the cylinder. This lowers the temperature of the air and hence the first-stage body and can cause any water inside the first-stage regulator to freeze, which can hamper the movement of the spring-operated first-stage valve. Some regulators have environmental kits that fill the space surrounding the first-stage spring with an antifreeze glycol or silicone solution. A diaphragm or rubber cap contains the antifreeze while still allowing the ambient pressure to be transferred to the first-stage mechanism.

The second-stage regulator can also freeze up in very cold temperatures. Any moisture in the second stage, including the moisture in exhaled air, can freeze, and the ice can jam the lever controlling the valve.

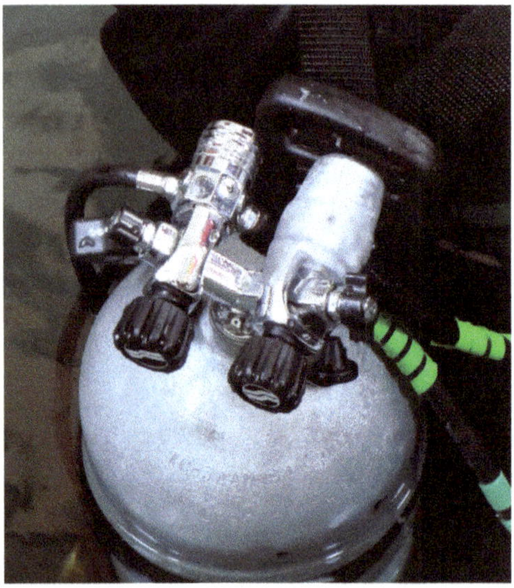

The Sherwood Maximus regulator has been shown to function extremely well in the sub-zero water temperatures in Antarctica. This is due to the design of the first stage, which has an overpressure bleed valve that keeps the freezing water from contacting the spring inside the regulator body. This regulator also has gold-plated fins in the second stage that capture the heat of the diver's exhaled air and conducts it to the second-stage mechanism, which prevents it from freezing.

Fig. 3.22 — A coating of ice may form on the first stage of a regulator due to the freezing temperatures.

To avoid regulator malfunctions, regulators must be cared for properly before, during, and after diving.

Regulators should be kept dry and warm before the dive. Be careful to avoid breathing on the regulator before submersion, except to briefly ensure it is functioning. The diver can inhale on the regulator and exhale after removing the regulator from the mouth. This will keep the moisture in the exhaled breath from freezing up in the second stage in very cold weather.

If the primary regulator freezes up and free flows during a dive, the diver should switch to the backup regulator and turn off the valve to the primary regulator to stop the free flow. Never use a regulator to fill a lift bag, as the rapid movement of air will usually cause a free-flow problem to develop.

After diving, take care when rinsing a regulator, especially if it is to be used again soon. Any freshwater remaining in the first or second stage can freeze up when exposed to cold ambient temperatures.

Tips for Keeping Water Out of Regulators

- Always open the cylinder valve briefly to blow out any moisture from the orifice before mounting the regulator.
- When purging the regulator for removal, hold the second stage lower than the first stage so that water cannot drip back to the first stage after the pressure has dropped.
- Remove the regulator carefully so ice or water cannot fall onto the filter of the regulator.
- Dry the dust cap thoroughly before attaching it to the regulator.
- The dust cap must fit snugly before rinsing the regulator.
- Do not depress the purge button while rinsing.
- Shake excess water from the second stage before hanging the regulator to dry.

Dive Knife, Mask, and Fins

A knife is mandatory equipment for each diver, as the potential for entanglement during ice diving is always present. Many divers prefer to carry a small, sharp knife to cut fishing line or other lines in which they might become entangled. Locate the knife in an area not subjected to suit squeeze, as this will cause straps to loosen and the knife sheath to move around. Many divers place the knife on the buoyancy compensator or the regulator console.

The type of dive mask used is not critical. It is best to avoid spitting into the mask for defogging, as this can freeze onto the inside of the face plate in cold weather. Commercial defogging agents work well for ice diving. Straps also can become brittle in cold weather, and spares should be available at the dive site.

The foot pockets of the fins need to be sufficiently large to accommodate the attached boots on most drysuits.

Instruments, Gauges, and Computers

Some electronic instruments will not function well in subfreezing temperatures. Liquid crystal displays may be slow to display due to the cold ambient temperature. Plastics can become very brittle and can shatter under freezing conditions, so take care to avoid rough treatment of instruments housed in plastic.

Batteries in dive computers and other instruments will also run low more quickly in cold temperatures. Carry spare batteries for models that allow user replacement.

Dive Lights

If the conditions are very dark under the ice, divers should use a minimum of two lights per diver. Small mini-lights are good for a backup in case of primary light failure. A powerful primary underwater light will brighten the way and make an ice dive more enjoyable. Several types of lights and batteries are available for different purposes.

A backup light should be compact and lightweight. Several flashlight-size models are available that weigh less than one pound. They will not have the intensity or beam angle of a larger light, but their advantage is in their compact size. A primary dive light is somewhat larger than a backup light. It will have greater power and a larger beam angle than smaller compact lights. They are also heavier and require more batteries. In darker conditions, some divers prefer to use a cave light, which has a separate battery canister and a high-powered light connected by a cable.

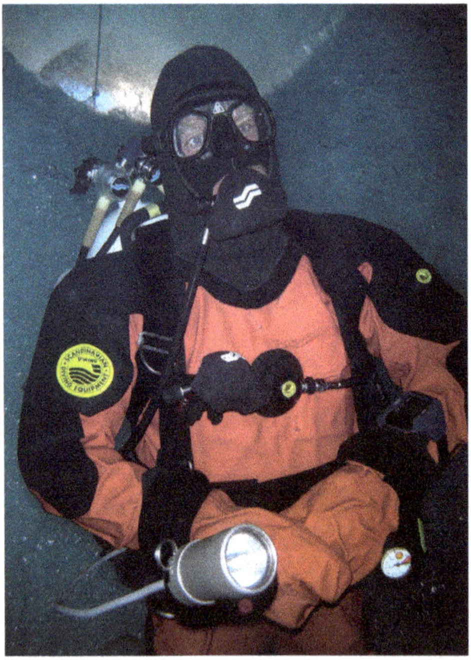

Attach a stretchable or adjustable lanyard to your dive light to prevent loss. The stretchable or adjustable feature is important so your hand can pull free in case the light becomes caught. Some lights float, and others sink. The ideal light for ice diving would be slightly positively buoyant and float with the beam pointing down. This would make it easier to recover if lost.

Chemical light sticks or a small single-battery marker light can be attached to your gauge console or cylinder valve to make it easy for you and your buddy to keep track of one another. They can also be used as a backup for signaling in case the primary light fails. The chemical light tube contains two separate chemicals. When the tube is bent, thin glass inside

Fig. 3.23 — Cave lights are high intensity and provide plenty of light under thick ice. (Photo courtesy of Henry Kaiser)

breaks and allows the chemicals to mix, which produces a glow that can last several hours. They are available in a variety of sizes and colors, which can be useful for identifying different groups of divers or dive leaders.

Surface-Supplied Diving

Surface-supplied diving, using a hose to deliver air and hardwire communications to the diver, is generally considered to be beyond the capabilities of normal recreational diving. However, it does have particular advantages when used for under-ice diving, such as the topside tender controls the primary and backup air supplies, and the presence of voice communications generally improves the safety of the dive.

As an intermediary between traditional scuba diving and the more commercial-oriented surface-supplied diving, some dive teams use tethered scuba diving. This is essentially a line-tended scuba diving mode utilizing full-face masks with communications and redundant scuba. This type of diving deviates from the traditional buddy diving concept of recreational diving and uses only one diver in the water at a time.

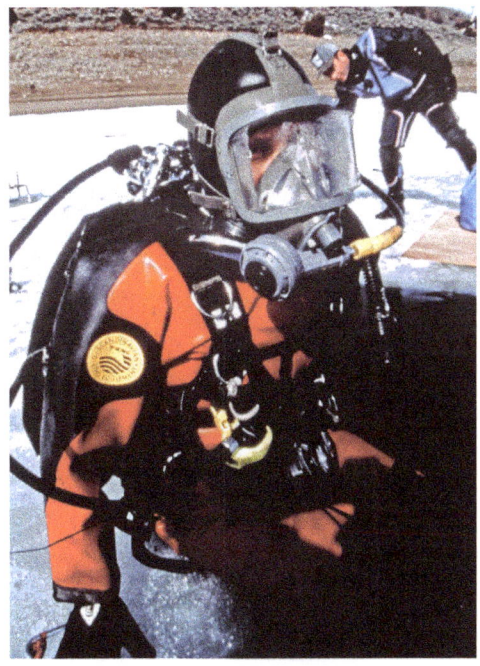

Fig. 3.24 — Full-face masks allow for communications and protection for the face.

It should be attempted only by those with proper training and equipment, such as rescue or scientific divers. Full-face masks can also be used with traditional scuba and have the advantage of providing diver-to-diver and diver-to-surface communications as well as providing more thermal protection to the diver's face.

Safety Harness and Lines

An adjustable chest harness made of nylon webbing is used to attach a safety line to the diver. It is worn over the exposure suit and under the scuba unit. A locking carabineer connects the safety line to the harness.

A safety line is required equipment for all under-ice diving. It is used for line-pull communication signals with the surface tender, for relocating the entry/exit hole in low-visibility conditions, and for safety if a current occurs during a dive.

The safety line should be constructed of strong synthetic material such as polypropylene or nylon and should be approximately 1/4 inch (7 mm) in diameter. Another

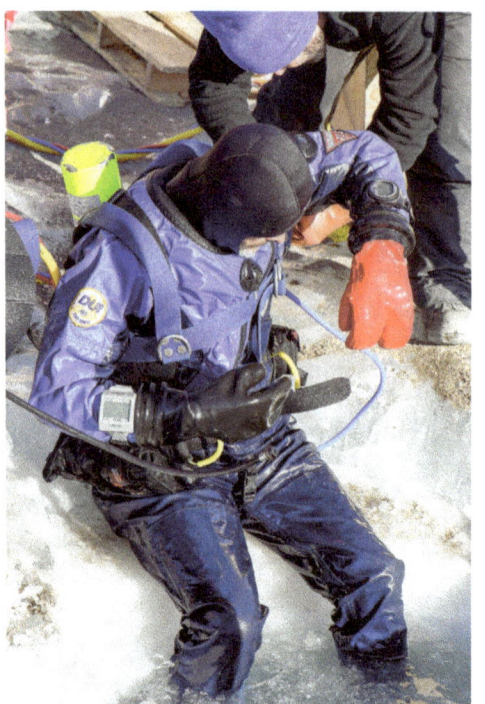

Fig. 3.25 — A chest harness with D-ring attachment points (Photo © Dale T. Andersen, all rights reserved)

commonly used line is 3/8 inch (10-11 mm) nonfloating polypropylene. Kernmantle rope is constructed of a high-strength inner core surrounded by an abrasion-resistant outer sheath. The heavier the line, the more drag and difficulty the diver will have in manipulating it and giving and receiving signals when it is extended. Thin lines tend to tangle more easily. Brightly colored line is available and easy to see underwater.

Some ropes have better abrasion resistance, which will increase the useable life of the line. Some lines are coated to prevent water absorption, which keeps the lines lighter in weight. Ropes are also prone to deterioration by ultraviolet sunlight and certain chemicals (see Table 3.1).

The safety line should be no longer than 150 feet (45 m) and marked off in

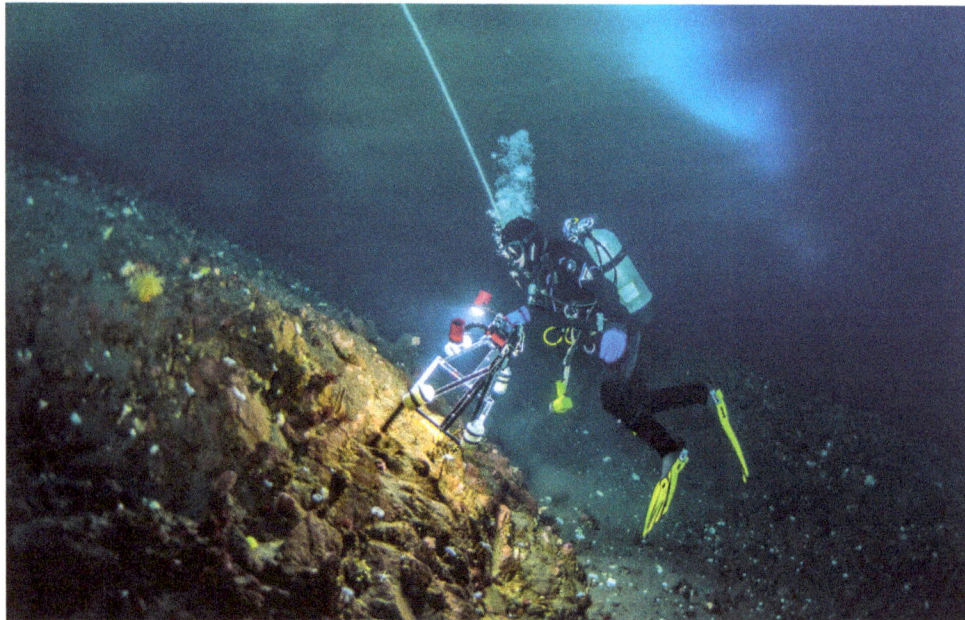

Fig. 3.26 — The diver must properly manage the safety line underwater and be responsive to line-pull signals from the tender. (Photo courtesy of Dale Stokes)

Table 3.1 Line materials, strength, and resistance to chemicals and U/V sunlight

Type of Line	Strength	Resistance to Oils/Greases	Resistance to U/V Sunlight
Nylon	Strongest most resilient	Very good to good	Good
Polyester	Strong Resilient	Very good to good	Good to excellent
Polyolefins (polypropylene)	Strong Moderate resilience	Very good	Fair. UV inhibitors can be added
Polyethylene	Lowest of all synthetics	Good to very good	Fair. UV stabilizers can be added
Manila	Low strength /weight ratio	Poor	Fair

increments of 25 feet (8 m). The marks can be made with tape and permanent markers or with cable ties. Store the line in a rope bag or five-gallon plastic bucket to keep it dry and free from entanglement. Ideally, store the line in a dry, dark area long term. Inspect lines periodically for signs of wear, which are characterized by fading, brittleness, crumbling fibers, abrasion, or cuts.

This loop is secured to the diver's safety harness using a locking carabineer. Secure the other end of the safety line at the surface to an ice screw or other stationary object that will not be moved and that cannot wear or sever the line.

The standby diver will use a floating type of line, usually made of polypropylene. It should be a bright color different from the diver's lines and at least 50% longer than the diver's lines.

Take care to avoid allowing line to become frozen by leaving it lying on the ice, which can weaken the line. It is also important to avoid stepping on the lines. It should be played in and out of the storage container (i.e., stacked or flaked) as the diver ascends and descends.

Thermal Protection for Surface Personnel

Ice-diving operations entail many hours of labor on the surface, ranging from hard work shoveling, digging, and sawing, to stationary standing while tending a diver underwater. The weather conditions can range from relatively mild to very cold with wind or snow. For these reasons, surface personnel should be equipped with warm, waterproof clothing. By layering clothing, one can adapt to the range of conditions and level of activity. There are many excellent synthetic fabrics such as polypropylene, Capilene, and others that can be worn next to the skin to wick away moisture from the body. Another layer of wool, sweaters, or synthetic insulating materials such as Thinsulate, Qualofil, or pile can be worn next, followed by waterproof yet breathable outerwear shell pants and jacket made of Gore-Tex, Thintech, or Ultrex. Down is very warm yet loses its insulative value when wet, which is likely when working around water and ice.

A good pair of waterproof boots with liners is essential for working on the ice. Waterproof overboots or gaiters can also be used to keep the boots dry. Crampons can be attached to the boots to facilitate walking on slippery ice.

A couple pairs of gloves or mittens with wool or synthetic liners are a must. The gloves will get wet when handling lines and dive equipment, and keeping an extra pair warm in an inside pocket is essential. Remember that tenders will be touching a lot of metal parts, which conduct heat away from the hands and can be dangerous if handled with bare hands. A great deal of heat can be lost through the head, and a balaclava or hat made of synthetic material or wool should be worn. Sunglasses should be worn if the tenders will spend long periods in bright conditions on the snow and ice. Sunscreen use is also recommended.

Emergency Equipment

Depending upon the location and circumstances of the dive, you will need to decide what type of emergency equipment to have on-site and what you will rely on rescue personnel to provide. Some type of communications equipment must be on-site or nearby, including a telephone or mobile radio. It is wise to have oxygen and personnel trained in its use at the dive site. Precious minutes can be lost waiting for rescue personnel to arrive. A standard first aid kit and extra blankets or a sleeping bag are also a necessity.

Additional Equipment

In addition to all the equipment discussed above, additional equipment may be required. Surface personnel should consider wearing a personal flotation device (PFD) in case of accidental water immersion. Dive lights and photographic equipment require fresh batteries or recharging and should be kept warm during diving preparations. Batteries lose their power much more rapidly at lower temperatures.

Some mountaineering equipment may be required depending upon the dive site. An ice ax or pick is handy for evaluating ice conditions and for use when walking or hiking on ice, especially if there are any slopes to be negotiated. Ice screws are useful for securing safety lines to the ice if no other strong, immovable object is

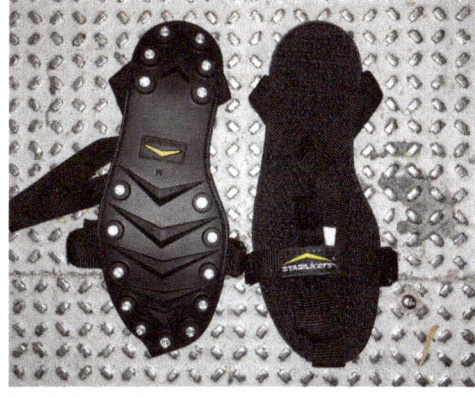

Fig. 3.27 — Studded crampons can be strapped over boots to prevent slipping on ice.

located nearby. Hollow, tubular ice screws or snargs are desirable as they can be placed into the ice with a minimum of ice displacement or shattering. Ice is displaced into the center of the screw as it is placed. Ice pitons can be driven into the ice and used as well. Locking carabineers are useful for securing lines to the diver. Shovels, tarps, and pallets are also useful. All of this equipment can be transported to the dive site on a sled or toboggan, which can be pulled behind people or towed behind a snowmobile.

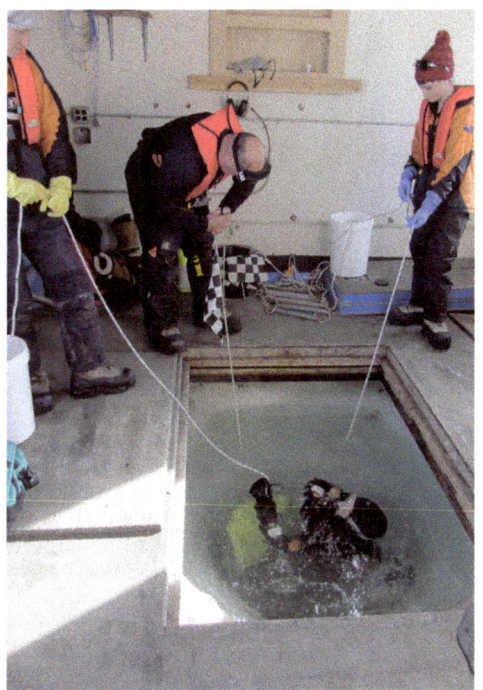

Fig. 3.28 — Surface tenders should consider wearing PFDs in case they fall into the water.

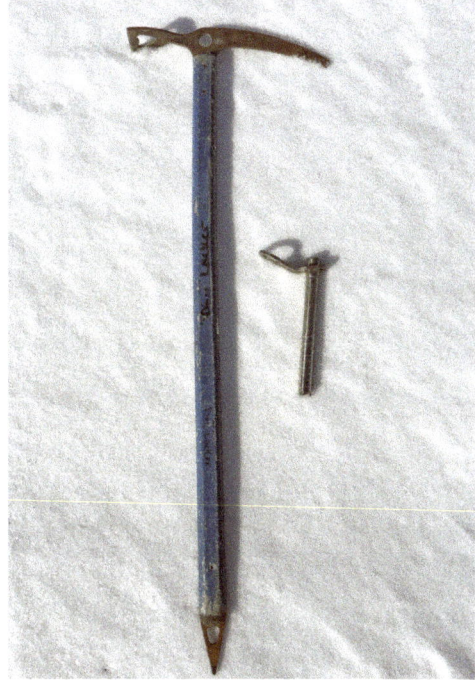

Fig. 3.29 — An ice ax (left) and ice screw (right) are useful for ice-diving operations.

CHAPTER 4
Ice-Diving Operations

Ice diving is an incredibly time- and labor-intensive activity. It takes a relatively large group of people and a considerable amount of time to find a suitable diving location, evaluate the ice conditions, prepare the site, review the dive plan, conduct the dive, and pack up to leave the site.

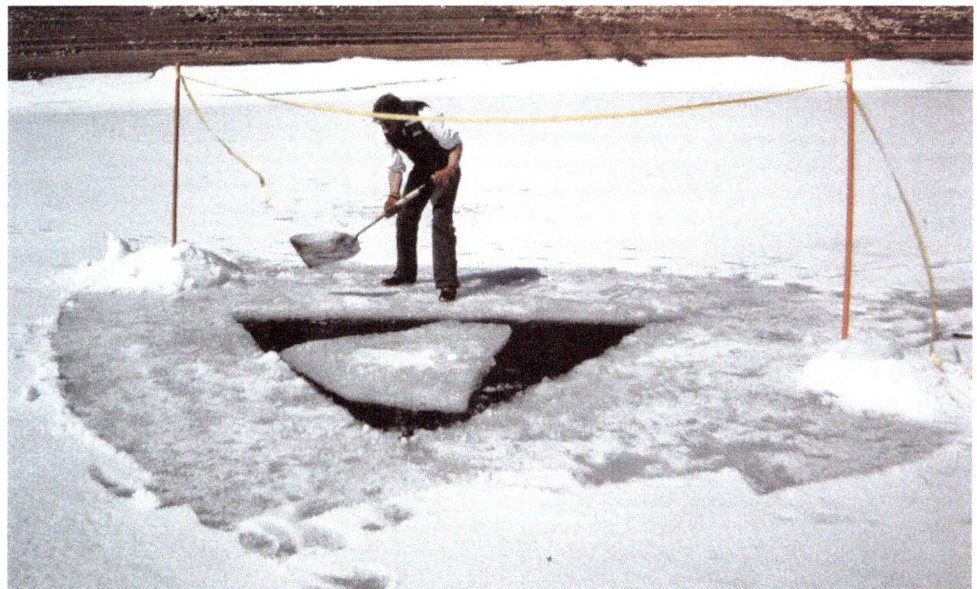

Fig. 4.1 — Ice diving requires considerable preparation before the dive.

Evaluating Ice Conditions

For ice-diving operations, the ice must be of sufficient thickness and strength to support the entire dive team and possibly vehicles or snowmobiles as well. A minimum thickness of 6 inches (15 cm) is required for small groups. Vehicles should be driven only onto ice of at least 12 inches (30 cm) thickness. New early-winter ice or older spring-melt ice may be particularly weak. Use caution when venturing onto this type of ice.

Two people are required to evaluate the ice conditions. One should be dressed in a drysuit, equipped with a harness and safety line, and have an ice pick or ice ax. This person will advance slowly onto the ice followed by the safety person, who is well behind. Ice thickness can be measured using an auger (drill) or ice pick. Some groups use gasoline-powered posthole-digging augers (4 inch or 10 cm diameter). A graduated marked measuring staff with a bent tip can be inserted through the hole and hooked under the ice so that an accurate measurement of ice thickness can be made. The ice thickness should initially be measured close to shore, as ice is often thickest near shore. If it is of sufficient thickness, then the team can carefully venture out to the anticipated dive location.

In marine situations, the fast-ice cover creates a wave-free and surge-free location for diving. However, cracks and pressure ridges are often in the ice due to tidal action and currents.

These cracks can be used with caution to gain access to the water. In pack ice, the broken ice cover eliminates the need to open an access hole. However, this type of ice is unstable and can move quickly with changing surface conditions. The surface tenders and divers must constantly monitor conditions for safety.

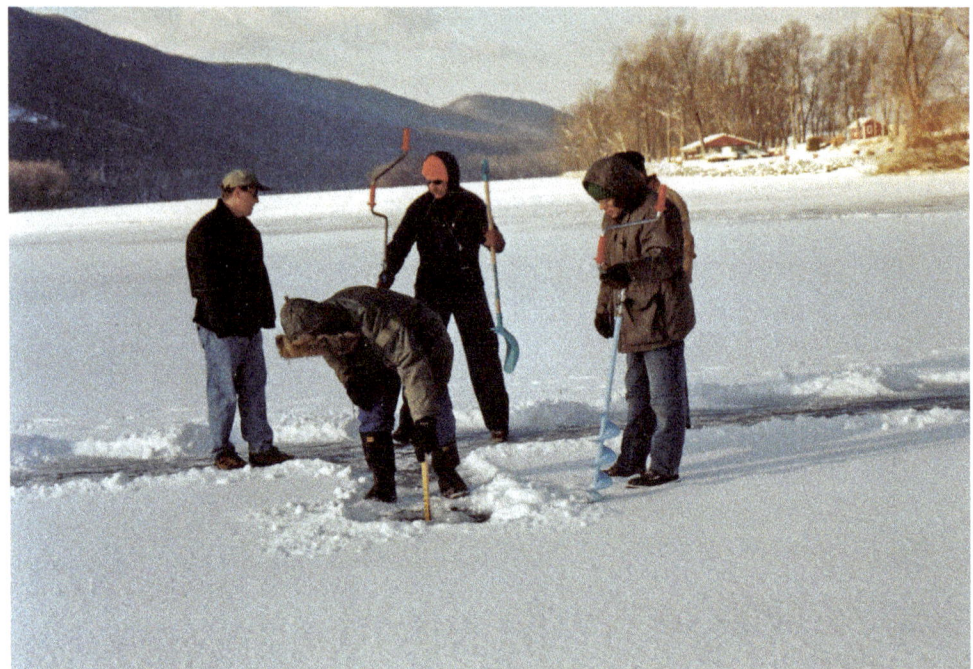

Fig. 4.2 — Measuring the thickness of the ice after drilling a test hole with an auger drill (Photo courtesy of Frank Morrow)

Preparing the Site

Once the ice thickness has been measured, it is a good idea to measure the bottom depth. This can be done by lowering a measured shot line with a light lead weight to the bottom.

Some type of surface shelter is also desirable to provide heating and shelter from the wind and elements. This can be in the form of a van, trailer, cabin, or tents. To minimize the chance of slipping on the ice, you can sprinkle sand or gravel around the dive hole area. Surface personnel and divers will stay warmer if their boots are not in contact with the ice. Sheets of plywood or insulating pads can be used for this purpose.

There are a number of different ways to gain access to the water through the ice. If the ice is relatively thin (up to about 3 feet or 1 m), the ice can be cut by hand using a

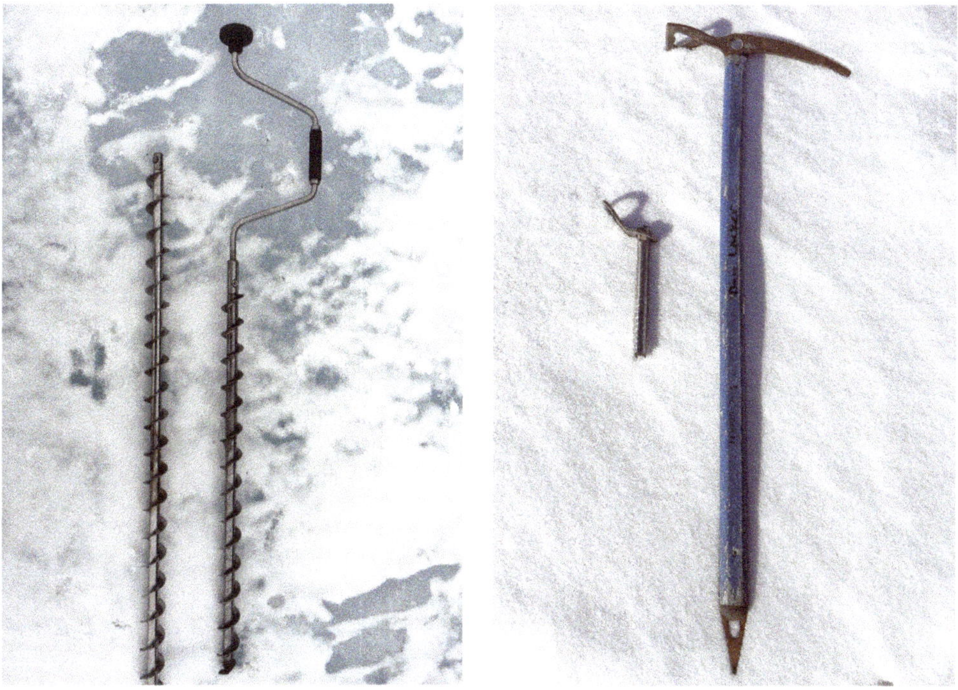

Fig. 4.3 — An ice drill with extra flights (left) that can be attached for thick ice, and an ice screw and ice pick ax (right)

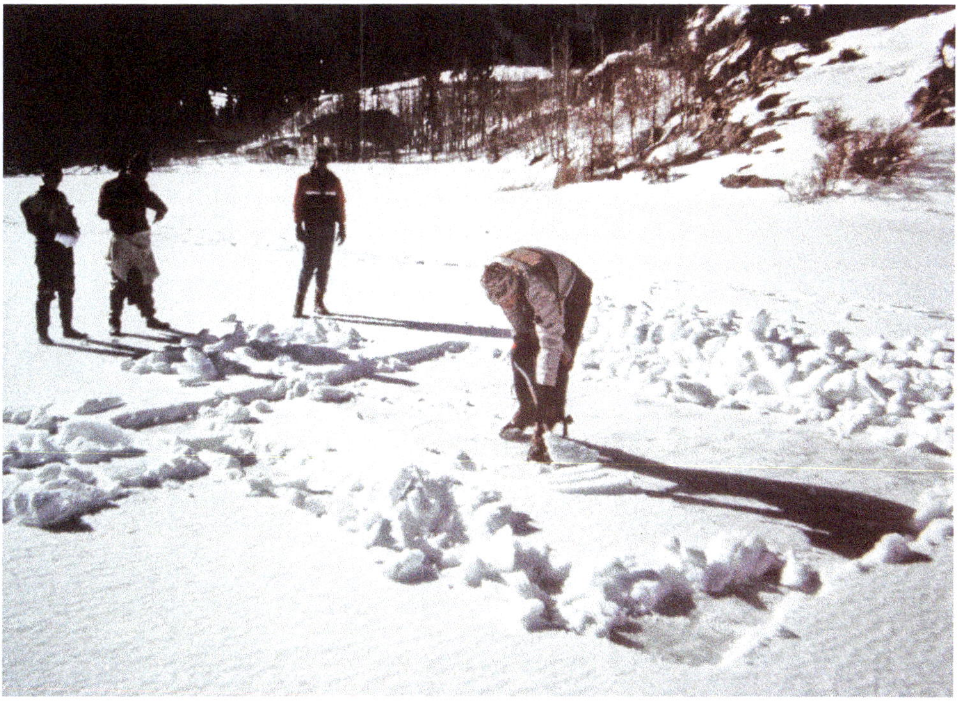

Fig. 4.4 — Once the site has been selected, the snow is shoveled off before cutting the ice.

Cold Water Diving   Ice-Diving Operations | 47

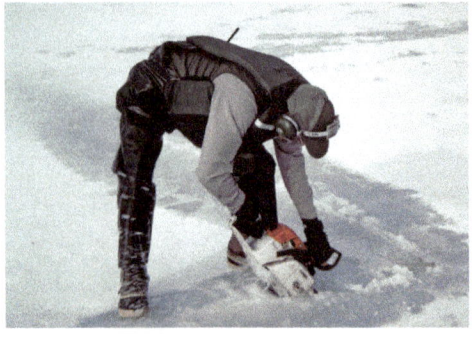

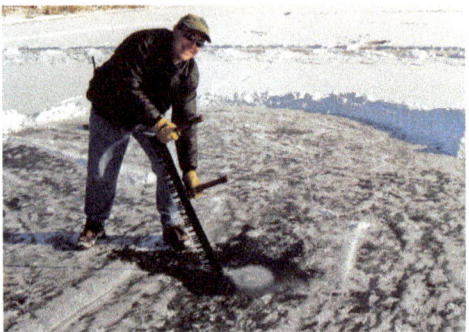

Fig. 4.5 — The ice can be cut with a chainsaw (top) or a handsaw (bottom). (Bottom photo courtesy of Frank Morrow)

handsaw, pick, or chainsaw. It is helpful to move the hole-cutting equipment to the dive site in a toboggan or on a sled rather than carrying it.

There are several options regarding the shape of the dive hole. Most divers use a triangular hole, as this requires one less cut than a square or rectangular hole. The corner angles also make it comfortable for entries and exits. The size of the hole should be large enough to accommodate two divers and a safety diver at the same time. This requires a hole of about 5 to 6 feet on a side.

The actual cutting of the ice requires the use of handsaws, breaker bars/chippers, and/or chainsaws. Surface personnel should wear waterproof clothing to minimize getting wet and cold. It is easiest to drill the corners of the hole with an auger and then cut from corner to corner

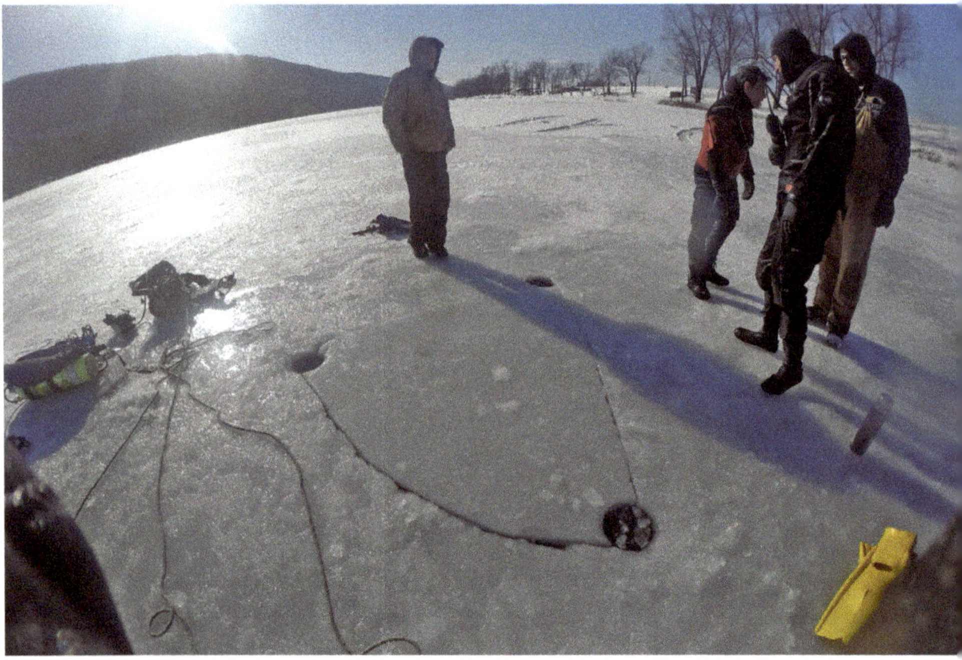

Fig. 4.6 — A triangular-cut block of ice with holes at the corners facilitates removal. (Photo courtesy of Frank Morrow)

through about 90% of the ice with a chainsaw to minimize splashing water onto the operator of the chainsaw. The actual cut into the corner holes and through the remaining ice is done last by hand with the ice saw or the chainsaw.

Ice is extremely heavy, and removing it from the hole can be difficult. Some dive teams place an ice screw in the center of the ice block and attach a line to it. The ice block can then be pushed under the surrounding ice to keep it safely away from the hole during the diving operations. The line allows for replacement of the block after the diving is completed. Another method is to drill a hole through the ice about 8 feet from one side of the triangle, drill another through the center of the ice block, and drill one more on the edge. The block can be pushed under the ice, lining up the holes, and a rod with a line attached can be pushed through both holes in the ice, securing the block to the frozen ice surface. A line can be passed through the extra hole on the edge of the block to pull it back into the hole at the end of the dive day.

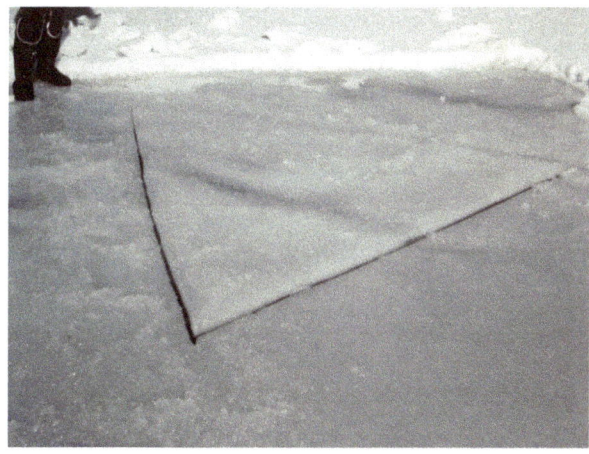
Fig. 4.7 — Once cut, the dive hole can be opened up by pushing the ice block under the ice.

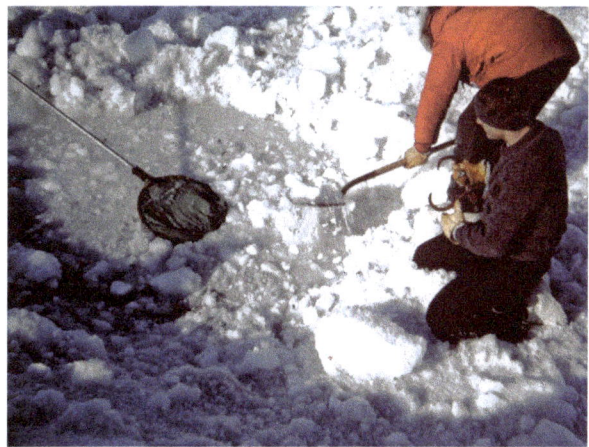
Fig. 4.8 — The dive hole then can be cleaned with a dip net, shovel, and/or ice tongs.

Some divers prefer to open one or more additional safety holes that can be used by divers in an emergency. All holes in the ice should be clearly marked so that surface personnel and others will not fall into them. Bamboo poles with bright colored flags work well for this purpose. Floating anchor ice and platelet ice dislodged by divers can fill up a dive hole. Tenders must clear it using a dip net.

Underwater visibility can often be improved by removing snow cover from the surface of the ice. One method of aiding divers underwater in locating the dive hole is to shovel radiating lines from the hole much like spokes of a wheel. V shapes can be shoveled along each line pointing to the direction of the hole.

Chemical lights or small flashing strobe lights can be hung on a line underwater to help divers locate the hole while underwater. An effective method of diver recall is to place a piece of metal such as a shovel or iron bar in the water and strike it with a hammer.

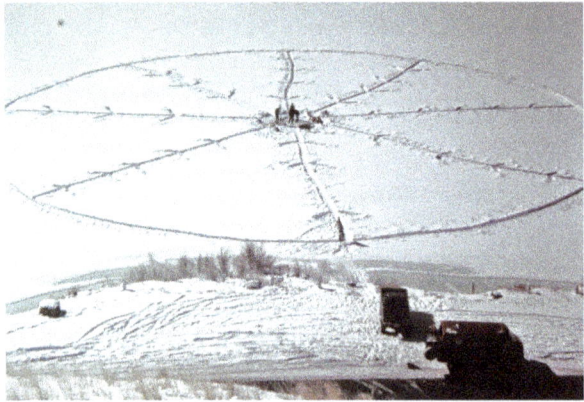
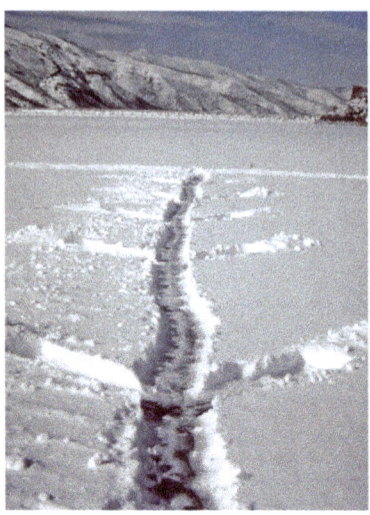

Figs. 4.9 — Spokes can be shoveled in the snow (above) to provide direction toward the hole to the divers below (right). (Photos courtesy of N. Langerman)

Dive Planning and Personnel

Ice diving requires extensive planning and a number of personnel to be done correctly. Before preparations for the dive begin, evaluate the weather conditions. A weather forecast will help determine if conditions are expected to deteriorate or improve. If the forecast or current conditions indicate bad weather such as heavy winds, an approaching storm, or extreme cold, postpone or cancel the dive.

Each diver should have a separate tether line and tender, but the divers must use care not to tangle the lines during the dive. As an alternative, one tender can control both divers using a Y line. This type of tether branches into a Y at the divers' end, with each diver having about a 6-foot length of line off the main tether.

The dive tender is one of the most important members of the diving operation. Preferably a trained ice diver, this person helps to assemble equipment and essentially dresses the diver into his equipment on the surface. While the divers are underwater, the tender pays out the safety line and maintains contact with the diver(s) by use of line-pull signals. The tender must keep in constant contact with the safety line while the divers are underwater. Tenders must stay warm to function well during the dive. Waterproof gloves, boots, and warm insulated clothing and headgear are essential for tenders. Some tenders use crampon spikes on their boots for more solid footing around the dive hole.

A safety diver must be suited up and ready to enter the water with little notice while divers are in the water. This diver usually has all equipment on and in place except for cylinder/buoyancy compensator, mask, and fins. The safety diver must be kept warm, and all equipment must be functional and ready to go if needed. An additional person is desirable to help with surface equipment and is especially helpful in an emergency to call for help, assist the safety diver, and assist divers in exiting the water.

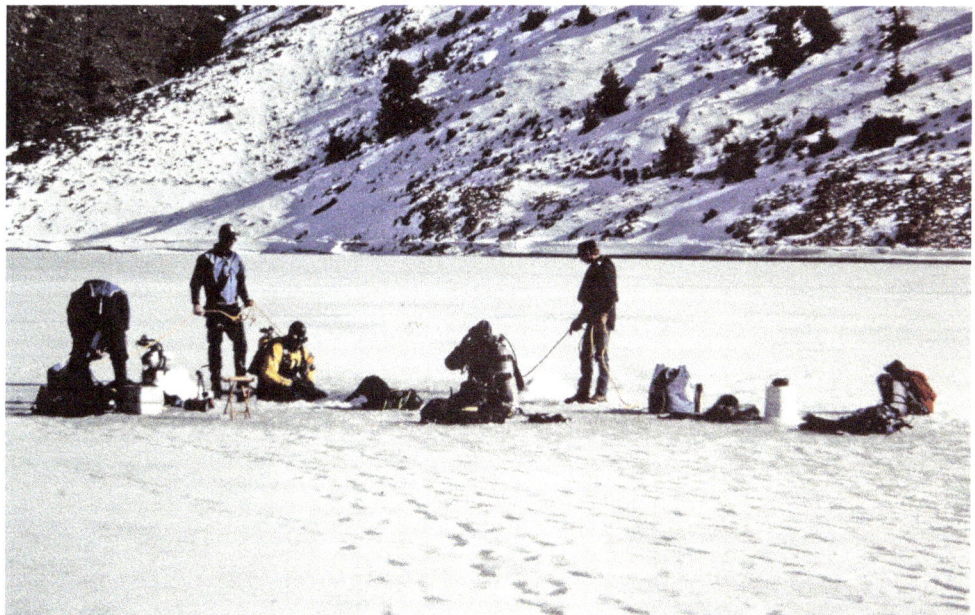

Fig. 4.10 — Dive planning and personnel are essential for proper ice-diving operations.

Table 4.1   Line-pull signals

Line-Pull Signal	Tender to Diver	Diver to Tender
1 pull	Are you OK?	I am OK.
2 pulls	Do you need more line?	I need more line.
3 pulls	No line remaining.	Take in slack.
4 pulls	Come up now!	Emergency! Pull me back!
Many repeated pulls		Help! Send safety diver!

Divers should discuss the dive plan before they suit up. Review line signals with the tenders. Signals should be simple and well understood by all participants. The tender should keep the line taut without hindering the diver's movements. A common rule is for the tender to give one pull every five minutes to check if everything is OK. Have a briefing with all personnel on site to review the objective of the dive, maximum depth and underwater time, tasks and responsibilities, distance to be traveled from the dive hole, any physical or biological hazards, and emergency procedures.

Diving at Altitude

Ice diving might be conducted at altitude, which may require additional planning due to the remoteness of the site, the terrain, and decompression and instrument calibration considerations. Sea-level decompression tables are generally useable only up to an altitude of 1,000 feet (330 m), and adjustments can be made depending upon the altitude (i.e., Cross Corrections). Some modern dive computers can detect changes in altitude and adjust the depth and time limits accordingly. Some can also be set to read depth in freshwater. Divers should complete training in altitude diving in open water before considering altitude ice diving.

Suiting Up

The divers should suit up in a place that is protected from the outside weather. Places such as inside a heated tent, motorhome, trailer, or cabin are all acceptable. This may be some distance from the actual dive site. A snowmobile or vehicle can transport divers to the dive site if necessary.

Keep all equipment warm before the dive — this is especially true for regulators, which can freeze up, especially in cold air conditions. Keep regulators dry, as any water in them can freeze in the cold air, causing a free-flow situation. If any regulators will be used on more than one dive during a day, keep them in warm water in an ice chest between dives.

The tender's duty before the dive is to assist the divers in donning their equipment, which allows the divers to wear their land gloves to keep their hands warm. When the divers have on their drysuits and are ready for diving, the tenders help them into their harnesses and weight belts. The divers then sit at the edge of the ice hole, where the tenders assist them with donning their buoyancy compensators, cylinders, gloves, fins, and mask; attaching the tether line to the diver's harness; properly routing and securing the regulators, including the redundant regulator; connecting all power inflators; and opening both cylinder valves (primary and redundant).

The diver's gloves are extremely important, as the hands tend to become cold first during a dive. If dry gloves are used, take care to ensure a correct seal on the cuff rings. Divers using wet gloves often have the tenders pour warm water from a thermos into the gloves prior to donning them.

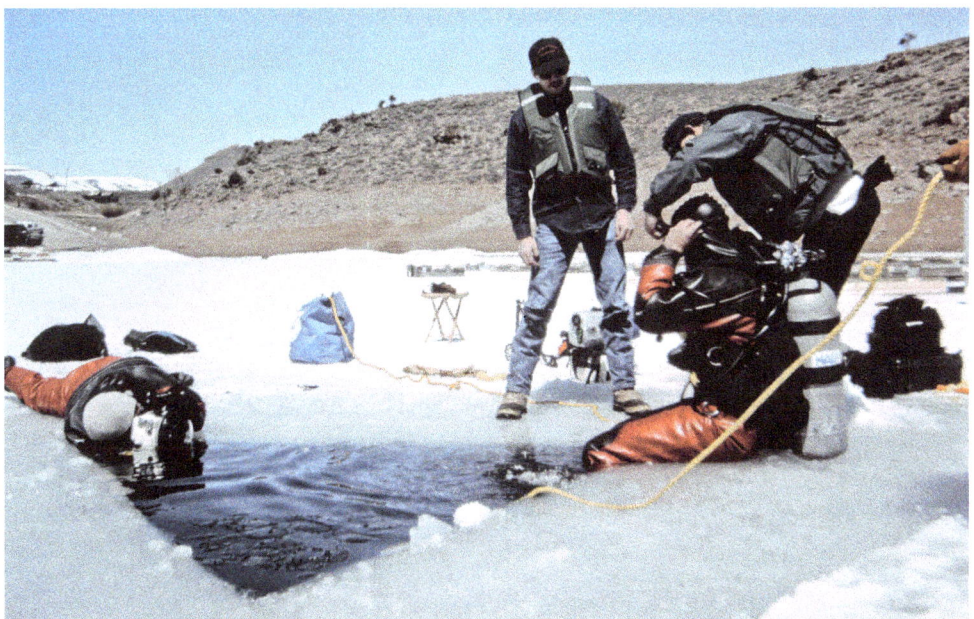

Fig. 4.11 — Tenders assist the divers in donning and adjusting all equipment.

As part of the final buddy check, the divers and tenders check that all of the equipment is properly placed and functional. One exception to this is the scuba regulator. It is important to take an initial breath to ensure proper function, but it is wise to not exhale through the regulator topside before the dive, as this can allow moisture to accumulate, which could cause a freeze up and free-flow situation. The divers should place the regulator in the mouth loosely just prior to entering the water and breathe around the mouthpiece until in the water. Once the regulator is immersed in the water, divers can breathe normally through it.

The Dive

The best entry to use is a seated entry at a corner of the hole, where the diver places both hands on one side and rotates around on the hands to slip into the water feet first. Both divers should descend slightly, test their regulators and lights, then descend together and maintain visual contact with each other. Add air to the drysuit only in short bursts of no more than one second to avoid a valve freeze up.

Avoid contact with the bottom, especially if it is silty, so that the sediment is not kicked up, thereby reducing the water visibility. The divers should also avoid crossing over each other's tether lines to avoid entanglement.

The tender and diver will communicate frequently using the line-pull signals shown in Table 4.1. The tender must always have control of the tether line during the dive. The diver should hold the line in one hand to feel the line-pull signals. All signals should be returned with an answering signal.

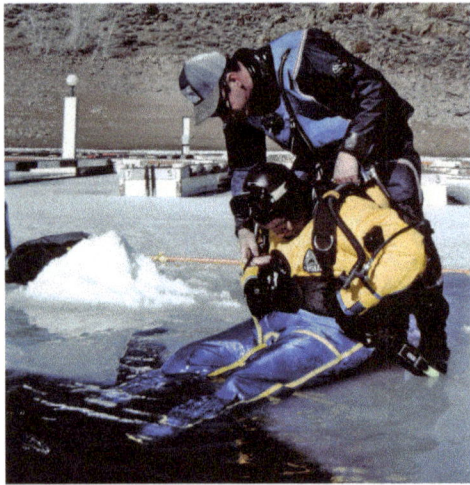
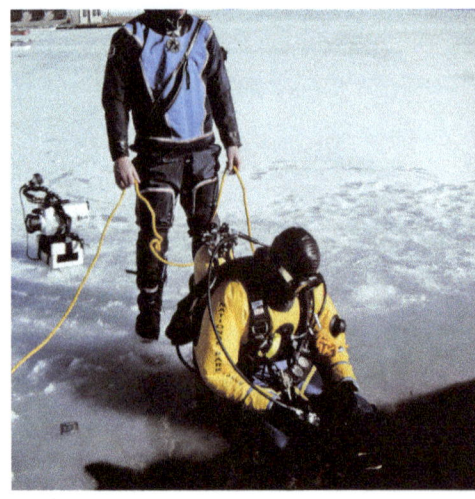

Fig. 4.12 — Tenders assist the diver before descent.

Fig. 4.13 — Entry can be made from a seated position on the ice.

The divers should descend to the predetermined maximum depth early in the dive and proceed to work their way shallower during the dive. The tenders will feed rope out of the rope bag as needed by the divers. A maximum distance of about 100 feet (30 m) from the dive hole is normally allowed. The divers should frequently monitor depth, underwater time, and gas pressure during the dive. The tenders will monitor surface weather conditions during the dive.

Gas management is critical in this overhead environment type of diving. The prudent diver will use the rule of thirds, in which one-third of the gas supply is used for descent and excursion to the maximum distance from the hole, the next third is used to return to the dive hole, and the remaining third is saved for emergencies. It is important to carry enough gas to breathe if the dive hole is lost and a safety diver must commence a search. Divers must also have a reserve supply of gas sufficient enough for the safety decompression stop.

Divers can become very cold while ice diving. With proper insulation under the drysuit, the body will stay quite warm. However, the hands and lips are usually the first areas to get cold. If

Fig. 4.14 — The tender communicates frequently with the diver via line-pull signals.

the lips become so cold that the diver cannot hold the regulator in his mouth, then he should hold the regulator in place manually and end the dive. The hands are also very susceptible to cold. If they become cold or numb to the point that dexterity is compromised, terminate the dive immediately.

Divers may become disconcerted if the visibility is less than the distance from them to the entry/exit hole. If there is any anxiety, then the divers should return to within sight of the hole. At the end of the dive, divers can ascend either diagonally by following the line back to the hole or horizontally along the bottom until underneath the hole and then making a vertical ascent. A safety stop of 3 to 5 minutes at a depth of about 15 feet (5 m) is recommended.

When the divers surface, they will often be cold and may be unable to manipulate their equipment efficiently. The tender should always assist the diver out of the water. Equipment such as weight belts or the BC and cylinder can be removed while the diver is in the water, if necessary. The tender may have to remove the low-pressure inflator hose from the drysuit. While one diver is removing his equipment and exiting the hole, the other diver should stay clear of the hole in case equipment is dropped. The divers should go to the warm shelter for rewarming and removal of the rest of the equipment, while the tenders secure the equipment and the area around the dive hole.

Surface personnel can switch places with the divers after everyone has had a chance to rest, warm up, and review the dive.

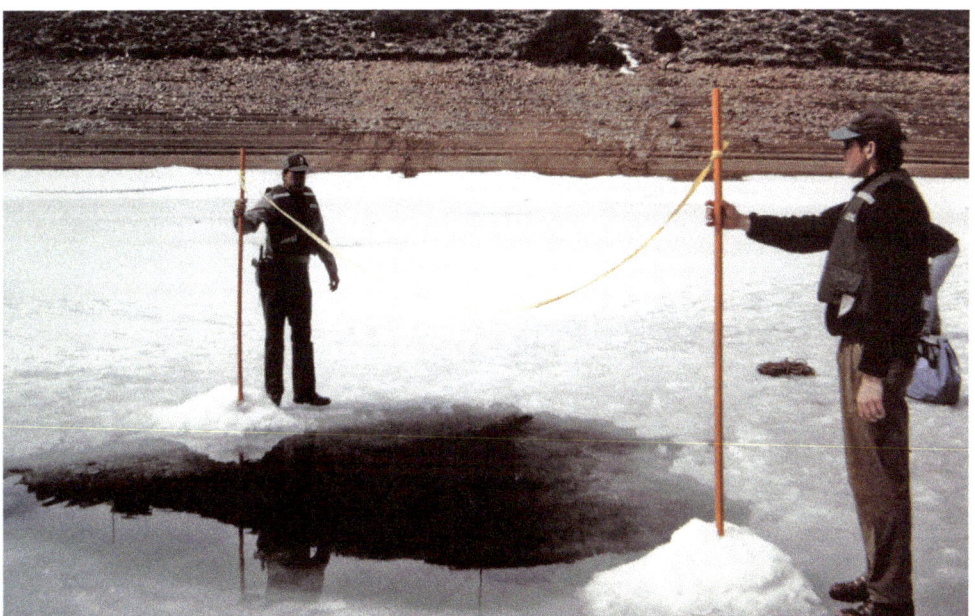

Fig. 4.15 — The site must be well marked before leaving it.

CHAPTER 5
Safety and Emergency Procedures

Safety is of paramount importance in all ice-diving operations. As in all types of diving, the prevention of problems is obviously preferable to having to solve them under adverse conditions. Emergency procedures should be practiced and be well understood by all participants in ice diving.

Environmental Hazards

Cold water and ice divers should evaluate and consider certain environmental hazards. Currents can be especially dangerous when diving in or under an ice cover. Establish the existence of a current by lowering a weighted line (about 2-3 lbs./1-2 kg.) into the water and checking for deflection in the current. Small streamers or flags can also be tied to the line to check for currents at various depths if the water visibility permits. Diving in currents greater than 0.5 knot (approx. 25 cm/sec) is not recommended.

Another potential danger of currents and wind in ocean ice-diving situations is moving ice. Small pieces of ice to large icebergs can pin divers to the bottom or block an exit point. Surface personnel must be attentive to moving ice and prepared to recall the divers to the surface if necessary.

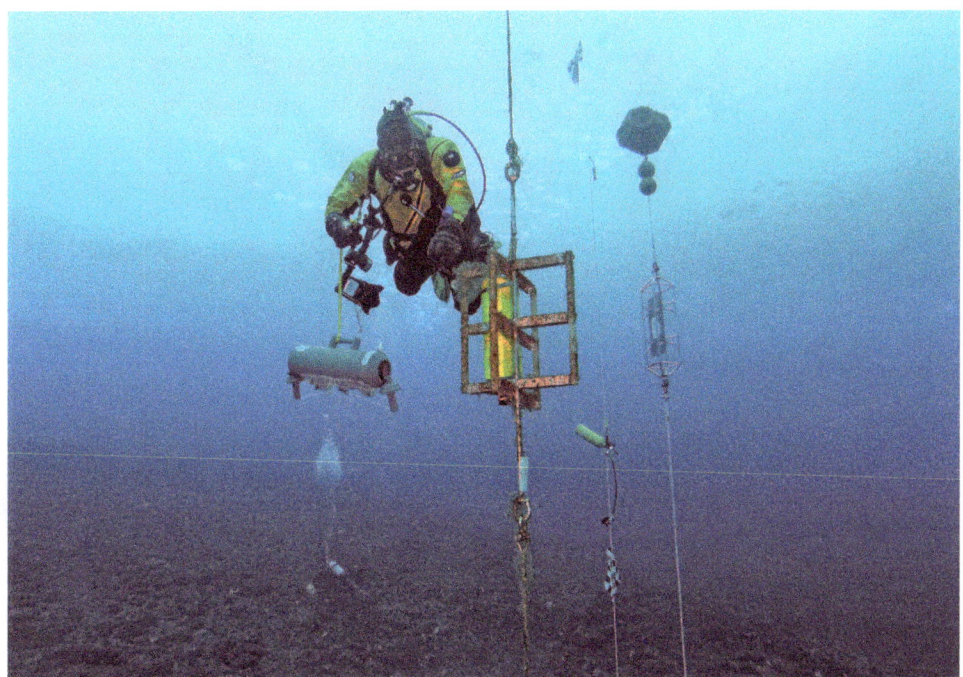

Fig. 5.1 — A weighted downline with flashing strobes, flags for evaluating current, and a bailout cylinder and regulator at the safety-stop depth

Blowing wind and moving ice are also extremely important when diving from a boat. Divers and boat drivers can become chilled easily when winds blow across ice and water. Have some type of insulation from the wind, such as a windproof overcoat or a sheltered cabin. Take care to ensure that moving ice does not block a safe passage back to shore.

Underwater visibility can be very good in some ice-diving conditions. It can range from spectacular 600-foot (180-m) visibility in the Antarctic, to 60-foot (18-m) visibility in some lakes, to zero visibility in plankton blooms, silty conditions, or where the ice is very thick and has considerable snow cover.

Diving within visual sight of the dive hole is comforting for most people. However, with a secure tether and communication with a buddy and surface tender, diving can continue beyond visual distance of the dive hole as long as other safety procedures are followed.

It is important for divers to avoid stirring up a silty bottom, which can reduce the visibility to zero. Proper buoyancy control and the use of a cave-diving type kick, with knees bent and fins up off the bottom, are essential to prevent silt from being resuspended in the water column.

Aquatic life is not much of a danger in ice diving. In certain marine situations, predators such as leopard seals or killer whales may present a problem.

Emergency Procedures

Regulator Freeze Up

Scuba regulators can freeze up in very cold conditions. To decrease this chance, keep regulators warm and dry before the dive. With the air temperature often lower than the water temperature, avoid breathing on the regulator on the surface, as this can easily promote freeze up and regulator free flow.

Never use a diver's regulator to fill a lift bag underwater. When large volumes of air are moved through the regulator, freezing and free flow can easily occur. For this reason, many divers attach the low-pressure drysuit inflator to the backup regulator to avoid placing excessive demand on the primary regulator first stage. The inflator can then be used even if the primary regulator and valve are turned off.

In the case of primary regulator freeze up or free flow, the diver should switch to the backup regulator, which should be attached to the buoyancy compensator or safety harness in a readily accessible location. After the diver establishes breathing, the diver or buddy should shut off the cylinder valve supplying the primary regulator and terminate the dive.

Inflator Valve Malfunction

Operate inflator valves only in short bursts, never more than a second or two at a time. Excessive use of the inflator can cause the mechanism to freeze. If the inflator valve becomes stuck open because of freezing or mechanical failure, air will be added rapidly to the suit. You should immediately disconnect the low-pressure inflator hose from the drysuit. Raise your arm to vent air from the suit, and manually depress the valve if necessary. If you are ascending, the volume of air in your drysuit will expand rapidly, especially in shallow water. If air is not venting fast enough from the exhaust valve, you can pull open your neck seat or a wrist seal while holding the arm above your head. This will dump air rapidly but will also allow some water inside the suit. Of course in a rapid ascent, you must exhale nearly continuously to avoid lung-overexpansion injuries.

If you cannot put air into the suit using the inflator valve, do not descend any further. You must terminate the dive. If you are neutrally buoyant, begin ascent. Use the BC as needed for additional buoyancy.

Dropped or Lost Weight Belt

If you feel your weight belt fall off your body, you should immediately try to grab hold of the belt. Depending upon the depth and your buoyancy, you may be able to kick hard toward the bottom to recover the weight belt. As long as you are holding onto the weights, you will not rise rapidly to the surface. Don and secure the weight belt. If you cannot recover the weight belt, try to grasp anything you can, such as kelp, a downline, rocks, etc. If you begin rising to the surface in an uncontrolled ascent, vent air out of the suit, and do a horizontal flare to slow the ascent rate. Practice these situations only under the supervision of a qualified instructor.

If you find yourself at the surface under the ice without a weight belt, it will be very difficult for you to maneuver your body. You can signal to the tender with your safety line to haul you in to the hole. You can assist by kicking with your fins and pushing off the ice with your hand. Your buddy should also be aware of your situation and can assist you as needed. As a last resort, the safety diver can be deployed and can easily follow the trapped diver's safety line to assist the buoyant diver back to the dive hole.

Entanglement

Ice diving typically involves tether lines, downlines, and other items that offer potential for entanglement. If a diver becomes entangled, the first consideration is to not panic. The diver or dive buddy can easily remove most entanglements. If you feel a line or other entanglement, remain calm, and do not spin around. Feel for the entanglement, and either gently remove it, or signal to your buddy for assistance. It may be necessary to cut free of an entanglement. Before cutting a line, be sure that it is not a tether line or other safety line used in the diving operation.

If a tender finds that a line feels tangled or gets no response from the diver via line-pull signals, then the standby diver must be deployed to investigate the situation. The safety diver can follow the line to the point of entanglement and remedy the problem.

Flooded Drysuit

A drysuit can become wet inside through minor leaks in the wrist or neck seals or through the zipper or other holes in the suit. Minor leaks are annoying but not necessarily hazardous. However, if the drysuit floods completely due to seal failure, zipper failure, or any other reason, terminate the dive immediately. Additional buoyancy for ascent may be required through use of the buoyancy compensator. Remove the drysuit immediately, and rewarm the diver.

Loss of the Dive Hole

One of the most serious things that can happen during ice diving is for the divers to lose the location of the entry/exit hole.

This would occur only if there was a loss of dive tether. If a diver notices that his tether line is lost, his first action should be to locate the line or the dive buddy. If the line is located, re-establish communication with the tender, reconnect the tether, and terminate the dive. If the line cannot be located, the diver should initiate physical contact with the buddy, and terminate the dive.

If neither the tether nor the buddy can be located, the diver should immediately ascend to under the ice ceiling and maintain a vertical posture with an arm extended over the head against the ice. This provides the largest possible target for a search procedure. The search procedure requires the safety diver to swim just under the ice in a circular pattern larger than the area the divers were estimated to be from the dive hole. The tether line should catch the lost diver. The lost diver should keep watch below him for the tether line if it passes by below him.

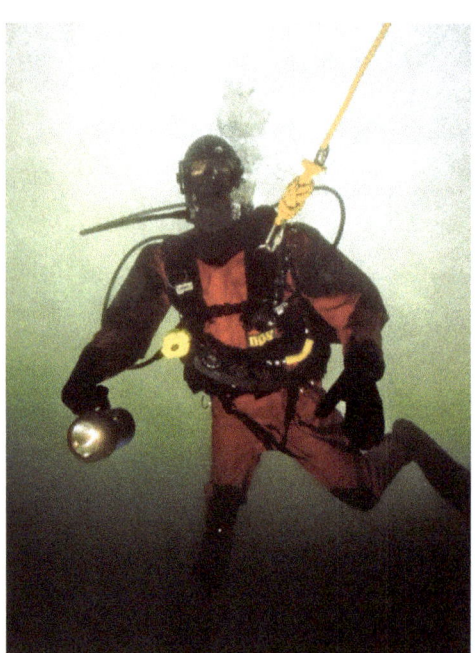

Fig. 5.2 — The tether line is the route back to the dive hole in low-visibility conditions. (Photo courtesy of J. Brooks)

If both divers become disconnected from the surface tethers, they should establish physical contact, ascend slightly, and slowly scan for the tethers in the water column. The divers may be able to retrace their path by following suspended sediments. If this does not produce results, the divers should surface and remain under the ice while the standby diver initiates a search like the one described above. The diver's air supplies will last much longer in shallow water. The surface tender will realize that the line(s) have gone slack and should

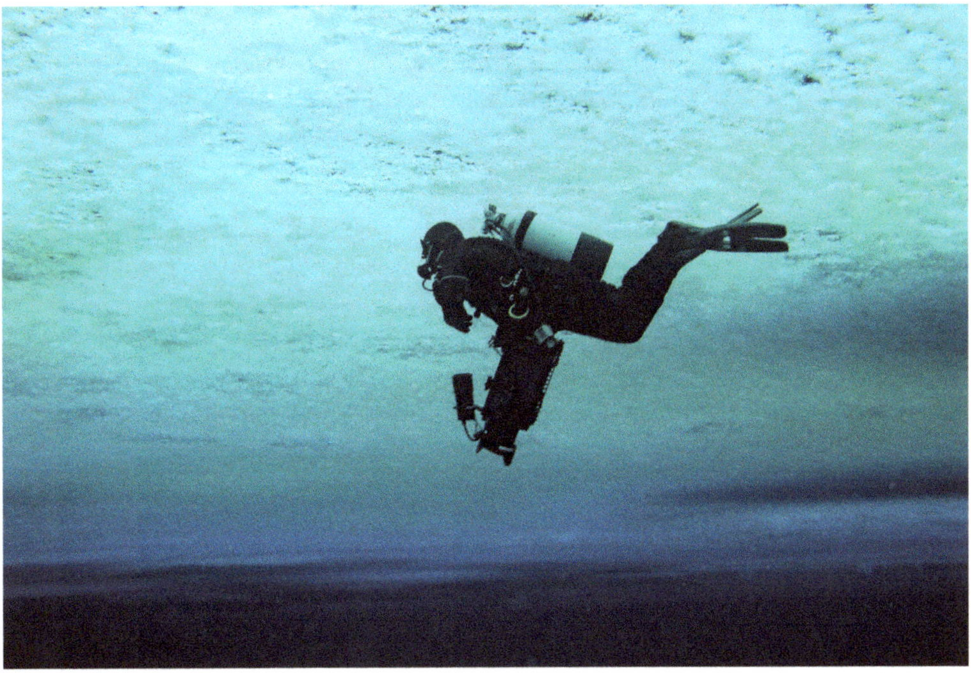

Fig. 5.3 — A lost diver under the ice ceiling provides a large search target for the safety diver. (Photo courtesy of Rob Robbins)

immediately lower a brightly colored downline, with strobe flashers if possible, to help the divers locate the access hole.

An alternate method for relocating the dive hole uses technology from cave diving. A lost diver could ascend to under the ice, secure the line from a gap reel to the underside of the ice using a piton or screw, and conduct a circle search for the dive hole in expanding circles. The diver would always be able to return to the starting point, and the standby diver could also accomplish the simultaneous search *(John Brooks, personal communication)*.

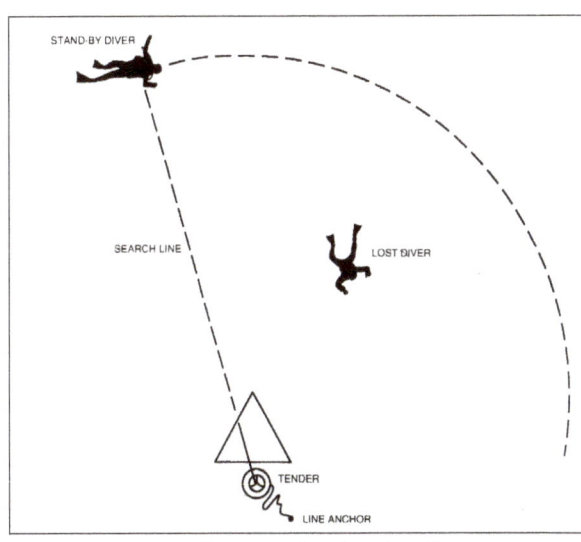

Fig. 5.4 — A safety diver searches for a lost diver.

Wind Chill

The dive team may encounter extremes of temperature on the surface during diving operations. The tenders must be prepared for cold temperatures, as the effectiveness of the surface personnel may affect the safety of the divers. The wind-chill factor can have an effect of much colder air on the skin (see Table 5.1).

People are especially vulnerable to sunburn at higher elevations. In addition, light is reflected from snow and ice, which makes areas such as ears, lips, and eyes particularly vulnerable to sunburn. Wear sunscreen and lip balm. Ultraviolet light is present even on cloudy days and can cause snow blindness. The basic symptoms of snow blindness are extreme pain in the eyes, sore scratchy eyelids, and headache. Treatment is to remove the victim to a dark place. Wear good-quality sunglasses to prevent this problem.

Table 5.1 Equivalent Wind Chill Temperature °F (°C)

Wind (mph)	Air Temperatures °F (°C)										
	40(4)	35(2)	30(-1)	25(-4)	20(-7)	15(-9)	10(-12)	5(-15)	0(-17)	-5(-21)	-10(-23)	-15(-26)
5	35(2)	30(-1)	25(-4)	20(-7)	15(-9)	10(-12)	5(-15)	0(-17)	5(-21)	-10(-23)	-15(-26)	-20(-29)
10	30(-1)	20(-7)	15(-9)	10(-12)	5(-15)	0(-17)	-10(-23)	-15(-26)	-20(-29)	-25(-32)	-35(-37)	-40(-40)
15	25(-4)	15(-9)	10(-12)	0(-17)	-5(-21)	-10(-23)	-20(-29)	-25(-32)	-30(-34)	-40(-40)	-45(-43)	-50(-46)
20	20(-7)	10(-12)	5(-15)	0(-17)	-10(-23)	-15(-26)	-25(-32)	-30(-34)	-35(-37)	-45(-43)	-50(-46)	-60(-51)
25	15(-9)	10(-12)	0(-17)	-5(-21)	-15(-26)	-20(-29)	-30(-34)	-35(-37)	-45(-43)	-50(-46)	-60(-51)	-65(-54)
30	10(-12)	5(-15)	0(-17)	-10(-23)	-20(-29)	-25(-32)	-30(-34)	-40(-40)	-50(-46)	-55(-48)	-65(-54)	-70(-60)
35	10(-12)	5(-15)	-5(-21)	-10(-23)	-20(-29)	-30(-34)	-35(-37)	-40(-40)	-50(-46)	-60(-51)	-65(-54)	-75(-60)
40	10(-12)	0(-17)	-5(-21)	-15(-26)	-20(-29)	-30(-34)	-35(-37)	-45(-43)	-55(-48)	-60(-51)	-70(-60)	-75(-60)

Little Danger | Increasing Danger | Great Danger

Frostbite

Windburn is similar to sunburn and is caused by cold wind blowing on unprotected skin, causing reddening and tenderness of the skin. Protect exposed skin from cold winds.

One result of exposure to cold temperatures is frostbite, which is the freezing of skin or the fluids in the tissues of the skin. The frozen area is usually small, and areas commonly affected are the nose, cheeks, ears, fingers, and toes. Signs and symptoms of frostbite include white or grayish-yellow skin color, pain sometimes intense, cold or numb feeling, and the appearance of blisters. These can progress to more serious symptoms such as mental confusion, impairment of judgment, and shock. It is critical to identify the early signs of frostbite and take protective action immediately.

First aid for frostbite includes covering the frozen part, keeping the victim warm, and rewarming the frozen area quickly by immersing it in a warm bath, no warmer than 105°F. Do not rub the area, as this can cause further damage. Loosely bandage the area with a dry, sterile dressing. Get medical attention as soon as possible.

Hypothermia

Prevention of hypothermia is of foremost concern to everyone involved in ice-diving operations. Hypothermia is defined as a lowering of the body core temperature to a stressful level. The central core consists of the brain, spinal cord, chest organs, abdomen, and pelvis. The peripheral shell consists of the limbs, muscles, and skin. The core temperature is regulated by the body to remain within narrow limits of the normal body temperature of 98.6°F (37°C), while the temperature of the shell can vary considerably. The skin temperature can be considerably lower than normal body temperature, which leads to vasoconstriction, which conserves the core temperature within normal limits.

The transfer of heat occurs between two systems of different temperatures in contact with each other. The larger the gradient — that is, the greater the difference in temperature between two items — the higher the rate of heat transfer. One of the laws of thermodynamics states that energy (heat) will move from the higher temperature (human body) to the lower temperature (water).

Both surface personnel and divers can lose heat through breathing, insufficient thermal insulation, and lack of movement. A loss of as little as 1-2°F (0.5-1°C) can result in a loss of mental capacity of 10-20% and as great as a 40% loss of memory. An individual with no thermal protection suddenly exposed to very cold water will often experience immediate disabling effects. As immersion occurs, there is a sudden involuntary inspiration or gasping response that may lead to inhalation of water. This response continues for one to two minutes with an extremely rapid breathing rate that the victim cannot control. As time progresses, muscle strength decreases, accompanied by pain and mental disorganization, with fear and panic reaction developing.

If the individual has some thermal protection, the immediate effects will not be as severe. Exercise or shivering will increase heat production by increasing the activity of skeletal muscle, but the agitation of water by activity increases heat loss.

Exercise increases the heat loss much more at low water temperatures and always increases the rate of body heat loss. It is not necessarily futile to try to stay warm with exercise, however. While exercise in the water causes heat loss to the water, you won't always get colder by exercising in the water, contrary to popular belief.

As chilling progresses and the core temperature fades, the individual will show predictable effects that loosely correspond to the core temperature.

Initial symptoms of hypothermia include sensation of cold, shivering, increased heart rate, urge to urinate, and slight incoordination in hand movements. Symptoms will progress to include increasing muscular incoordination, stumbling gait, slowing or cessation of shivering, weakness, apathy, drowsiness, confusion, and slurred speech. In severe hypothermia, where the core temperature is 85-90°F (29-32°C), shivering stops, and the person is unable to walk or follow commands, complains of loss of vision, and has confusion progressing to a coma. At a core temperature of 65-85°F (18-29°C), symptoms are muscle rigidity, decreased blood pressure, lowered heart rate and respiration, dilated pupils, and a dead appearance.

There is some evidence that short-term adaptation can be achieved by individuals in cold climates. A study of divers in the subarctic found improved vasoconstriction, which led to a reduction in thermal conductance by the tissues over a 45-day period.

Management of Heat-Loss Victims

Suspecting the existence of hypothermia is the first step in management. Chilling may be mild with little risk to the individual or severe with a possibility of death. The mildly chilled individual will be awake, complaining of cold, possibly shivering, and able to converse intelligently. The moderately chilled individual will be awake but may be confused, apathetic, or uncooperative, and may have difficulty with speech. If severely chilled or hypothermic, the victim may be unconscious with a slow heart rate and respiration or may even appear dead with no detectable heartbeat. The victim who is moderately or severely hypothermic may be made worse or placed in cardiac arrest by careless attempts at rewarming. Hypothermia is an emergency in slow motion, and improper handling may actually create a fatal outcome. The cold heart is especially sensitive, and victims who are alive when found may develop cardiac arrest if handled roughly during the initial evaluation and transportation. The rescuer must transport and rewarm the victim without precipitating cardiac arrest.

Rewarming is of extreme importance, of course, but should not be attempted unless it can be done properly. However, it sometimes becomes necessary to rewarm a chilling victim in an area far from medical care. The first attempts should use passive methods, including protection against further heat loss by removing wet clothing and covering in layers. Remember to provide layers between the victim and the ground or deck and to cover the head, which is a major source of heat loss. The fully alert and cooperative victim may be given warm liquids to drink; this will deliver negligible amounts of heat but will help to correct any dehydration. Strictly avoid coffee, tea, caffeine drinks, and alcohol. Oral fluids may include balanced electrolyte solutions such as Gatorade, Gastriolyte, or Infalyte, which are available in powder form. If the victim is awake, do not exercise him/her because muscular activity will bring cold blood from the periphery to the core. The mildly or moderately chilled victim will soon return to a near normal temperature.

Immersion of the victim in a hot bath is thought to be risky unless limited to the trunk only, with the extremities left out. Similarly, body-to-body contact is limited to bare skin in the trunk area only. Current research indicates that the victim will not have increased cooling of the heart on immersion, limbs and all, in a hot bath.

The severely hypothermic victim may be unconscious or appear dead. Look carefully for signs of life such as breathing, movement, or a pulse at the groin or in the neck over the carotid artery. If breathing or movement is present and the heart is beating, then CPR is not needed. If the breathing rate is six or less per minute, then very gentle mouth-to-mouth breathing at a slow rate may be started while being extremely careful to avoid rough handling of the victim.

If there are no signs of life, start CPR and make arrangements for emergency transport to the nearest medical facility. Rewarming of the severely hypothermic victim cannot be accomplished in the field. Continue CPR until emergency assistance arrives, if possible. There have been successful resuscitations after prolonged CPR, in part because of the protective effect of hypothermia.

Preventing chilling requires training, judgment, and experience. The diver must understand the use of external insulation to conserve body heat and must be able to control heat loss. Recreational divers sometimes encounter very cold conditions in ice diving or winter diving in deep quarries and lakes. All ocean dives are in water below body temperature. Wetsuits provide some degree of thermal protection depending on the style, material, and thickness, but they become compressed with increasing depth and lose much of their insulating properties. The "woolly bear" or open-cell undergarment worn under a drysuit is effective but also compresses and loses some insulation value. If wet, the "woolly bear" loses practically all of its insulating value. Type B marine Thinsulate is an alternative that retains insulation value when wet.

The diver should be prepared for the actions to be taken once in the water. These include efforts to minimize heat loss, such as remaining still and assuming the H.E.L.P. position (heat escape lessening position). This position is assumed by drawing the knees up to the chest and holding them with crossed arms. The position is unstable and not easy to achieve without practice, as one tends to roll forward or backward. Consequently, it is good to practice the position from time to time. The huddle position with other persons — in which everyone wraps arms around one another and pulls into a tight circle, remaining as still as possible — is surprisingly effective in conserving heat.

Conscious Diver with Lung Overpressure or Decompression Illness

Pulmonary barotrauma accidents can be a result of rapid ascent without exhalation. This can occur in ice-diving situations in which proper buoyancy is not maintained because of freezing inflator mechanisms or the loss of a weight belt. Signs and symptoms include difficulty breathing, pain in the chest, and, in severe cases, disturbed vision, unconsciousness, or paralysis.

Decompression illness (DCI) can occur after dives supposedly within the "safe" limits of decompression tables or dive computers or as the result of a rapid ascent. It is wise to plan dives in advance with adequate safety margins, to ascend slowly according to the specified rate for the tables or computer used, and to perform a precautionary stop for at least three minutes at a depth of 15 feet (5 m).

Signs and symptoms include pain in the joints, skin rash, nausea, weakness, and, in severe cases, unconsciousness and paralysis.

The field first aid treatment for these situations is the same: Keep the diver warm and on his back, administer CPR as needed, and provide 100% oxygen. Make arrangements for transportation to a medical facility.

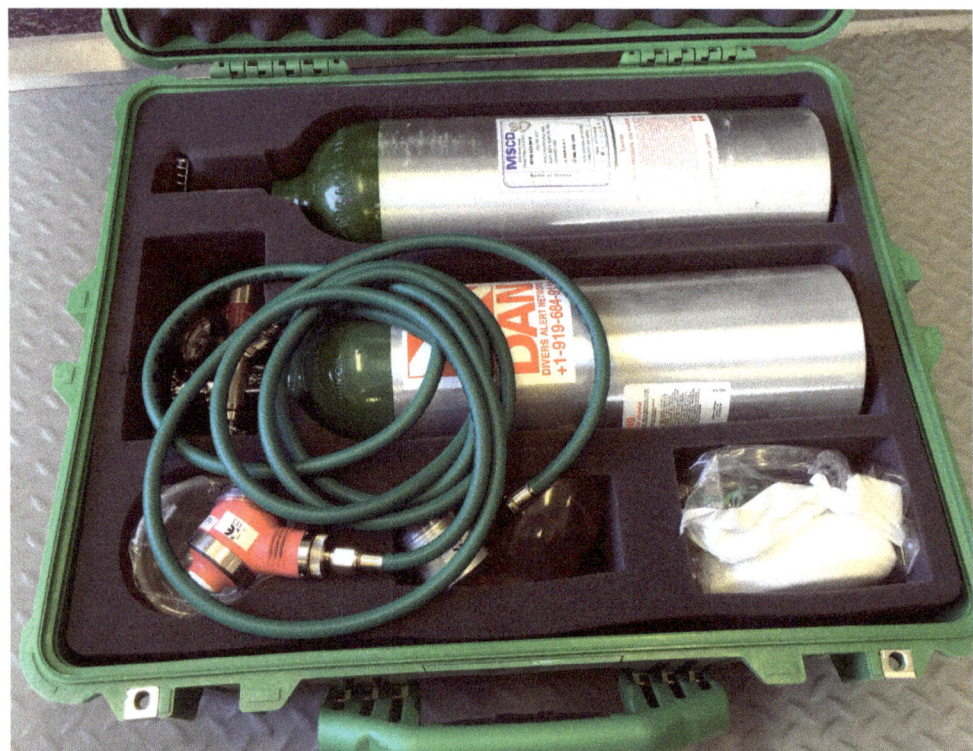

Fig. 5.5 — Oxygen should be available on-site to treat diving emergencies.

Unconscious Diver

An unconscious diver underwater is an extremely serious situation. Rescue procedures are similar to those for open-water situations except for the presence of the tethers and overhead ice. The buddy should signal to the surface immediately with more than four pulls on the tether line. The buddy should make contact with the unconscious diver, shake him, turn him to a face-up position if necessary, and establish a do-si-do position. If the regulator is in the victim's mouth, leave it there. It may be necessary to release the weight belt of the victim to establish sufficient buoyancy for ascent. However, use caution, as excessive positive buoyancy may be realized on ascent, causing potential danger to victim and rescuer alike. It is probably best to attempt ascent with the weight belt left in place. If the diver was neutrally buoyant or close to it at depth, then ascent should be relatively easy, and indeed air will have to be vented from each diver's suit on ascent. The safety diver may be able to assist with positioning the victim and venting air on ascent.

At the surface, the tenders will assist in removing the diver from the water. Summon emergency help immediately. Remove the cylinder and weight belt from the diver, who is placed in a horizontal position on his back. Check for breathing. Initiate artificial respiration and CPR, if necessary. If the victim is in a hypothermic state, breathing and pulse rates may be very slow, so give sufficient time and care to check for vital signs. Remove the drysuit from the upper torso to properly perform CPR. Administer oxygen if required. Shelter the diver from the cold, preferably in a heated place.

Depending upon the location of the dive site and the nearest medical treatment facilities, a diver may have to be evacuated by helicopter. The importance of having a well-thought-out emergency plan in remote locations cannot be overstressed.

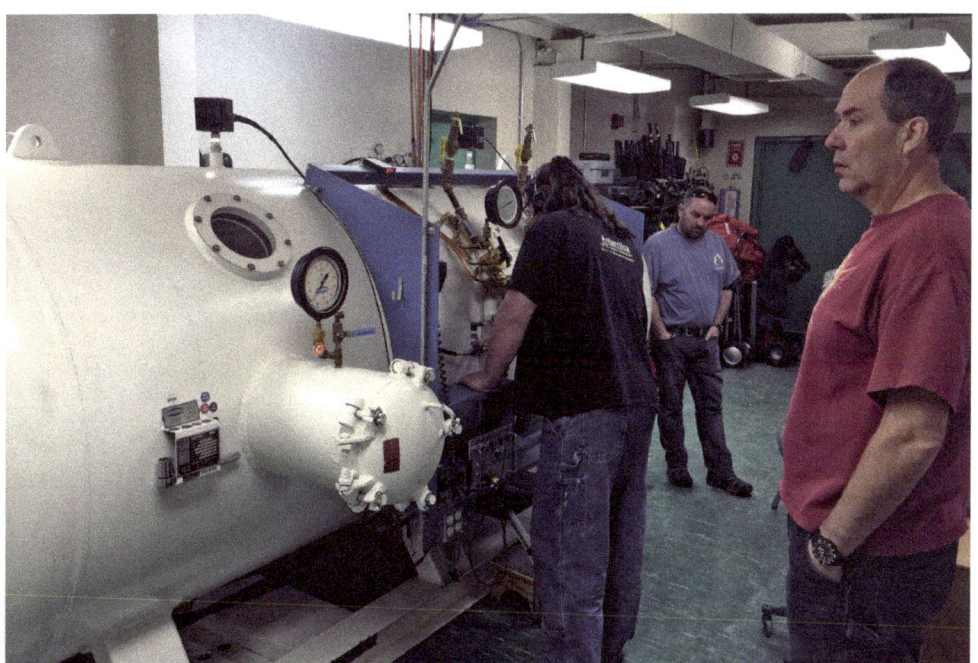

Fig. 5.6 — A recompression chamber may not be immediately available to ice divers. Seek medical evaluation at the nearest hospital or clinic. The staff there can provide intermediate treatment and initiate a timely transfer to an appropriate and available hyperbaric facility if needed.

Summary

Ice diving is a potentially dangerous activity, therefore safety is of paramount importance. An emergency plan should be developed, reviewed, and practiced in simulation. It is important to recognize that rescue operations may be hampered by weather, cold, and remote locations. The best policy is prevention of accidents.

References

American Red Cross. *Standard First Aid*. St. Louis, MO: Mosby Lifeline. Available from: www.redcross.org

Barsky SM. *Diving in High-Risk Environments*. Fort Collins, CO: Dive Rescue Inc. International; 1990.

Barsky SB, Heine JN. Observations on flooded dry suit buoyancy characteristics. In: Lang M, ed. *Advances in Underwater Science '88: Proceedings of the American Academy of Underwater Sciences Eighth Annual Scientific Diving Symposium*. Costa Mesa, CA: American Academy of Underwater Sciences; 1988:1-11.

Barsky SB, Long D, Stinton B. *Dry Suit Diving: A Guide to Diving Dry*. San Diego, CA: Watersport Publishing; 1992.

Bright CV. *Diving in the Arctic*. Nav Res Rev. 1972; 25(8):1-12.

Cinnamon J. *Climbing Rock and Ice: Learning the Vertical Dance*. Camden, ME: Ragged Mountain Press; 1993.

Dinsmore DA, Bozanic, JE, eds. *NOAA Diving Manual: Diving for Science and Technology*. 5th ed. North Palm Beach, FL: Best Publishing Co.; 2013.

Flemming NC, Max MD. *Scientific Diving: A general code of practice*. 2nd ed. Flagstaff, AZ: Best Publishing Co.; 1996.

Gloersen P, Campbell WJ, Cavalieri DJ, et al. 1992. *Arctic and Antarctic Sea Ice, 1978-1987: Satellite Passive Microwave Observations and Analysis*. Washington, DC: Scientific and Technical Information Program, National Aeronautics and Space Administration; 1992.

Haddock SHD, Heine JN. *Scientific Blue-Water Diving*. La Jolla, CA: California Sea Grant College Program; 2005.

Harbin MA, Mastro J, Bozanic J, et al. *Antarctic Scientific Diving Manual*. Englewood, CO: Antarctic Support Associates; 1994.

Heine JN. *Advanced Diving: Technology and Techniques*. St. Louis, MO: Mosby Lifeline; 1995.

Heine JN. *Diving Dry: Skills and Techniques*. Montclair, CA: National Association of Underwater Insturctors, Mosby-Year Book; 1995.

Heine JN. *Scientific Diving Techniques: A Practical Guide for the Research Diver*. 2nd ed. Palm Beach Gardens, FL: Best Publishing Co.; 2011.

Hendrick W. The parameters of safe ice diving. *Sources*. 1994 March; 37-40.

Hendrick W, Zaferes A. *Ice Diving Operations*. Tulsa, OK: PenWell Corp.; 2003.

Jenkins WT. *A Guide to Polar Diving*. Panama City, FL: Naval Coastal System Laboratory; 1976.

Lamb IM, Zimmermann MH. Benthic marine algae of the Antarctic Peninsula. In: Pawson DL, ed. *Biology of the Antarctic Seas V*. Washington, DC: American Geophysical Union; 1977:130-229.

Lang MA, Sayer MDJ, eds. *Proceedings of the International Polar Diving Workshop*. Washington, DC: Smithsonian Institution; 2007.

Lang MA, Stewart JR, eds. *Proceedings of the American Academy of Underwater Sciences Polar Diving Workshop*. Costa Mesa, CA: American Academy of Underwater Sciences; 1992.

Long R. Dive suit buoyancy control problems and solutions. In: Egstrom G, Lang M, eds. *Proceedings of the Biomechanics of Safe Ascents Workshop*. Costa Mesa, CA: American Academy of Underwater Sciences; 1990:103-110.

Madigan DL. Sunlight degradation of rope. *National Safety News*. 1984 March; 129(3):54-56.

Mastro J, Pollock N. Regulator temperature and performance during Antarctic diving. Draft report, American Academy of Underwater Sciences; 1995

McMullen J. *The Basic Essentials of Climbing Ice*. Merrillville, IN: ICS Books; 1992.

Mercer S. *Antarctic Diving Manual*. Christchurch, NZ: New Zealand Antarctic Programme; 1992.

Neushul M. Diving in Antarctic waters. *Polar Record*. 1961 January; 10(67):353-358.

Neushul M. Diving observations of sub-tidal Antarctic marine vegetation. *Botanica Marina*. 1965; 8(2-4):234-243.

Palmer R. *An Introduction to Technical Diving*. Middlesex, England: Underwater World Publication; 1994.

Peckham V. Year-round scuba diving in the Antarctic. *Polar Record*. 1964 May; 12(77):143-146.

Rey L, ed. *Arctic Underwater Operations: Medical and Operational Aspects of Diving Activities in Arctic Conditions*. London: Graham and Trotman Ltd.; 1985.

Skreslet S, Aarefjord F. Acclimatization to cold in man induced by frequent scuba diving in cold water. *Journal of Applied Physiology*. 1968 Feb.; 24(2):177-181.

Somers LH. *The Cold Water Diver's Handbook*. Ann Arbor, MI: University of Michigan Press; 1991.

Stinton R. Dry suit exhaust valve performance: effect on buoyancy control and rate of ascent. In: Egstrom G, Lang M, eds. *Proceedings of the Biomechanics of Safe Ascents Workshop*. Costa Mesa, CA: American Academy of Underwater Sciences; 1990:111-122.

Index

air, 2, 4, 6, 8, 9, 10, 15, 17, 21, 26, 27, 28, 29, 32, 33, 35, 34, 36, 37, 39, 52, 53, 58, 59, 60, 62, 67
   consumption, 21
   management, 15, 18, 21, 39, 54, 60
   temperatures, 4, 6, 8, 10, 36, 37, 38, 52, 58, 62
Alaska, vii, 2, 79
altitude diving, 9, 14, 52
American Academy of Underwater Sciences (AAUS), 79
anchor ice, 49
ankle weight, 33
Antarctic, vii, ix, 2, 3, 7, 58
   US Antarctic Program, ix
Antarctica, vii, 2, 36, 79
antifreeze, 36
Arctic, 2, 3, 7
auger, 15, 45, 46, 48
austral, 8
ax, 43, 45, 47

BC. *See* buoyancy compensator.
backup, 2, 35, 37, 38, 39, 58
   air supply, 39
   lights, 38
   regulator, 2, 35, 37, 58
boots, 14, 27, 31, 34, 37, 42, 46, 50
brine channels, 2, 10
bubbles, 9, 35
bubbly ice, 9
buoyancy, 14, 15, 16, 17, 18, 22, 23, 24, 26, 32, 33, 37, 51, 52, 58, 59, 60, 65, 66, 67
   compensator, 17, 24, 33, 37, 51, 52, 58, 60
   control, 15, 16, 17, 18, 58
   systems, 14, 32
buoyancy compensator, 17, 24, 33, 37, 51, 52, 58, 60
buoyant, 38, 59, 67

California, 6, 79
Canada, 7
Canadian, 2
Capilene, 42
carabineer, 39, 41, 43
ceiling, 1, 60, 61
chainsaw, 15, 48, 49
chemical light sticks, 38, 39, 50
clear ice, 9
cold, vii, ix, 1, 2, 4, 6, 7, 8, 10, 14, 15, 21, 27, 28, 36, 37, 38, 42, 48, 50, 52, 54, 55, 57, 58, 62, 63, 64, 65, 67, 69
   water, vii, ix, 1, 2, 4-10, 14, 21, 27, 36, 57, 63, 79
   weather, 1, 14, 21, 37, 69

communication, 2, 14, 15, 16, 18, 39, 42, 50, 52, 53, 54, 58, 59, 60
   line-pull, 14, 16, 18, 39, 40, 50, 51, 53, 54, 59
   with tenders, 16, 18, 39, 50, 52, 53, 58, 59, 60
computers, 9, 38, 52, 66
confined water, 16
CPR, 65, 66, 67
crampons, 42, 43, 50
currents, 4, 6, 7, 10, 11, 15, 39, 46, 50, 57, 65
cutting, 13, 14, 47, 48, 59
   hole, 14, 48
   ice, 13, 47, 48
   line, 59
cylinder, 13, 14, 32, 35-36, 37, 38, 51, 52, 55, 58, 67
   bailout, 57
   pony bottle, 13, 36
   valve, 14, 35-36, 37, 38, 52, 58

DCI. *See* decompression illness.
D-ring, 40
decompression, 52, 54, 65, 66
   stop, 54
   tables, 52, 66
decompression illness, 65-66
dip net, 49
dive
   lights, 13, 14, 38-39, 43, 53
   plan, 14, 18, 45, 52
   planning, 1, 2, 14, 50-52, 66
   tender, 1, 14, 16, 17, 18, 29, 39, 40, 42, 43, 46, 49, 50, 52, 53, 54, 55, 58, 59, 60, 62, 67
diver rescue, 16, 19, 42, 64, 66, 67, 69
diving, vii, ix, 1-12, 13-19, 21-43, 45-55, 57-67, 69
   altitude, 15, 52
   Arctic, 2
   buddy, 39
   cave, 58, 61
   cold water, vii, 1-2, 4-12
   commercial, 2, 3, 39
   drysuit, 16, 17
   emergencies, 66
   equipment, 2, 3, 16, 21-43
   from a boat, 58
   ice, 1-12, 13-19, 21-43, 45-55, 57-67, 69
   in currents, 57
   in rivers, 10
   introduction to, 1
   location, 45, 46
   open-water, 13
   preparations, 43, 45
   recreational, 39
   research, 2

scientific, vii, 2
scuba, ix, 39
surface-supplied, 19, 39
winter, 65
double-hose regulators, 2, 3, 36
downlines, 13, 57, 59, 61
dry gloves, 28, 29, 52
drysuit, 2, 3, 4, 13, 14, 15, 16-17, 21, 22-23, 23-27, 27-29, 29-32, 32-33, 33-34, 34-35, 37, 45, 52, 53, 54, 55, 58, 59, 60, 65, 67, 79
   accessories, 27-29
   air volume in, 26, 32, 59
   boots, 27, 30, 37
   care and maintenance 17, 21, 33-34
   exhaust valve, 17, 23, 26, 27, 31, 59
   features of, 23-27
   flooded, 15, 33, 60
   gloves, 28, 29, 52
   hoods, 27, 28
   neoprene, 22, 29
      closed-cell, 22
      crushed, 22
   seals, 25, 26, 27, 28, 34
   self-donning, 24, 29
   service and repairs, 34-35
   shell, 23
      rubber, 23, 24
      trilaminate, 23, 24
      urethane-backed nylon, 23
   sizing, 27
   skills, 16-17
   storage, 34
   types of, 22-23
   training, 16
   undergarments, 14, 16, 21, 22, 23, 27, 29-32, 34, 65
   valves, 26, 27, 31, 33, 34, 53
   weight and buoyancy systems, 32-33
   zippers, 17, 23, 24, 25, 33, 34, 35, 60

electrolyte solutions, 64
emergency, 2, 13, 14, 15, 16, 17, 18, 42, 49, 51, 52, 57-67, 69
   equipment, 2, 13, 14, 17, 42
   evacuation, 16
   plan, 67, 69
   procedures, 15, 18, 52, 57-67
      conscious diver with lung overexposure or decompression illness, 65-66
      dropped or lost weight belt, 59
      entanglement, 59
      flooded drysuit, 60
      frostbite, 62-63
      hypothermia, 63
      inflator valve malfunction, 58-59
      loss of the dive hole, 60-61
      management of heat-loss victims, 64-65
      regulator freeze up, 58
      unconscious diver, 66
      wind chill, 62
entanglement, 15, 37, 41, 53, 59
entry, 2, 15, 18, 39, 53, 54, 55, 60
   hole, 2, 18, 39, 55, 60
   seated, 53, 54
   techniques, 15, 53
environmental hazards, 15, 57-58
environmental kits, 36
epilimnion, 4
equipment, ix, 1, 2, 13, 14, 16, 17, 21-43, 50, 51, 53, 55
   additional, 42-43
   communications, 42
   cylinders and valve configurations, 35-36
   dive knife, mask, and fins, 37
   dive lights, 38-39
   drysuit, 2, 3, 4, 13, 14, 15, 16-17, 21, 22-23, 23-27, 27-29, 29-32, 32-33, 33-34, 34-35, 37, 45, 52, 53, 54, 55, 58, 59, 60, 65, 67, 79
   emergency, 2, 13, 14, 17, 42
   hole-cutting. *See* equipment: ice-cutting.
   ice-cutting, 13, 14, 46-50
   instruments, gauges, and computers, 38
   malfunction, 1
   mountaineering, 43
   personal flotation device, 42
   photographic, 43
   regulators, 36-37
   safety harness and lines, 39-42
   strobe lights, 13, 50, 57, 61
   surface, 51
   surface-supplied diving, 39
   tender, 14
   thermal protection for divers, 21-35
   thermal protection for surface personnel, 42
exhaust valve, 17, 23, 26, 27, 31, 59

fall turnover, 4
fast ice, 10, 12, 46
first aid, 14, 16, 42, 63, 66
   field, 66
   first aid kit, 42
   frostbite, 63
fleece, 30, 31
floes, 10, 12
frazil, 10
free flow, 26, 33, 37, 53, 58
   inflator valve, 26, 33
   regulator, 37, 53, 58
freeze, 2, 8, 10, 37, 52
freeze up, 15, 16, 26, 33, 36, 37, 52, 53, 58, 59, 65
   inflator valve, 26, 33, 53, 58, 59, 65
   regulator, 15, 16, 36, 37, 52, 53, 58
freezing, 1, 2, 4, 7, 8, 9, 10, 33, 36, 38, 62

ocean waters, 7
seawater, 10
skin, 62
temperatures, 2, 4, 33, 36, 38
water, 1, 2, 8, 9, 33, 36
freshwater, 2, 4, 8-9, 14, 33, 37, 52
    ice, 8-9, 14
        bubbly, 9
        clear, 9
        snow, 9
    rinse, 33
frostbite, 14, 62-63
full-face masks, 19, 39

gas management. *See* air management.
Gastriolyte, 64
Gatorade, 64
gauges, 14, 38
gauntlet-style gloves, 28
glacial lakes, 9
gloves, 14, 27, 28, 29, 30, 31, 32, 42, 50, 52
    dry, 28, 29, 52
    five-fingered, 28
    gauntlet-style, 28
    heated, 30, 31, 32
    squeeze, 28
    undergloves, 28
    waterproof, 50
Gore-Tex, 42
grease ice, 10
Great Lakes, 8, 9
Gulf Stream, 7

H valve, 35
harness, 13, 14, 33, 39-40, 41, 45, 52, 58
hazards, 9, 10, 15, 52, 57-58
    biological, 52
    environmental, 15, 57-58
heated undergarments, 31, 32
history of ice diving, 2-4
hoods, 14, 27, 28
hypolimnion, 4
hypothermia, 1, 14, 21, 63-64, 65

ice,
    anchor, 49
    ax, 43, 45, 47
    bubbly, 9
    ceiling, 1, 60, 61
    clear, 9
    diving, 1-12, 13-19, 21-43, 45-55, 57-67, 69
    fast, 10, 12, 46
    floes, 10, 12
    freshwater, 8-9, 141

grease, 10
multiyear, 10
overhead, 1, 16, 21, 54, 66
pack, 10, 11, 46
pancake, 10, 11
polar, 10
saltwater, 14
screw, 13, 14, 41, 43, 47, 49, 61
sea, 10, 11
snow, 9
ice diving, 1-12, 13-19, 21-43, 45-55, 57-67, 69
    environment, 4-12
        freshwater ice, 8-9
        lake environments, 9
        rivers, 10
        sea ice, 10, 11
        seasonal thermal stratification in lakes, 4, 5, 6
        variation in ocean temperatures, 4-8
    equipment, 21-43
        additional, 42-43
        cylinders and valve configurations, 35-36
        dive knife, mask, and fins, 37
        dive lights, 38-39
        emergency, 42
        instruments, gauges, and computers, 38
        regulators, 36-37
        safety harness and lines, 39-42
        surface-supplied diving, 39
        thermal protection for divers, 21-35
        thermal protection for surface personnel, 42
    history of, 2-4
    operations, 45-55
        dive planning and personnel, 50-52
        diving at altitude, 52
        evaluating ice conditions, 45-46
        preparing the site, 46-50
        suiting up, 52-53
        the dive, 53-55
    safety and emergency procedures, 57-67
        conscious diver with lung overpressure or decompression illness, 65-66
        dropped or lost weight belt, 59
        entanglement, 59
        environmental hazards, 57-58
        flooded drysuit, 60
        frostbite, 62-63
        hypothermia, 63-64
        inflator valve malfunction, 58-59
        loss of dive hole, 60-61
        management of heat-loss victims, 64-65
        regulator freeze up, 58
        unconscious diver, 66-67
        wind chill, 62
    training, 13-19
        classroom curriculum, 13-16
        confined water, 16
        drysuit, 16

open water, 17-19
suggested drysuit skills, 16-17
Infalyte, 64
inflator valve, 15, 17, 26, 31, 33, 34, 53, 58, 59
    free flow, 26, 33
isothermal, 4

JIM suit, 3

K valve, 35
kernmantle rope, 40
knife, 14, 37

Labrador Current, 7
lake, 1, 4, 5, 6, 8, 9, 14, 58, 65, 79
    alpine, 8
    environments, 9
    freshwater, 8
    Great Lakes, 8, 9
    glacial, 9
    layers, 4, 6
    mountain, 9
    stratification, 4, 5
    visibility, 58
latex, 22, 23, 25, 26, 27, 28, 33, 34
    hoods, 28
    mitts, 27
    seals, 22, 23, 25, 26, 27, 28, 33, 34
lights, 2, 13, 14, 38-39, 43, 50
    backup, 38
    cave, 38
    chemical, 38, 50
    dive, 13, 14, 38-39, 43
    floodlights, 2
    marker, 38
    mini-, 38
    strobe, 13, 50, 57, 61
line-pull signals, 14, 16, 18, 39, 40, 50, 51, 52, 53, 54, 59
lines, 13, 14, 17, 37, 39-42, 43, 45, 46, 49, 50, 52, 53, 55, 57, 59, 60, 61, 66
    colored, 40, 41
    deterioration, 40, 41
    downlines, 13, 57, 59, 61
    floating, 41
    materials, 41
    safety, 13, 39, 40, 41, 43, 45, 50, 59
    shot, 46
    signals, 14, 16, 18, 39, 40, 50, 51, 52, 53, 54, 59
    storage, 41
    strength, 41
    tether, 14, 50, 52, 53, 59, 60, 66
    weighted, 57
    Y, 50
lost dive hole, 16, 54, 60-61

lost diver, 16, 17, 19, 60-61
lung overexpansion, 59
lung overpressure, 65-67

metalimnion, 4
mittens. *See* mitts.
mitts, 2, 14, 27, 28, 29, 42
    latex, 27
    three-fingered, 28
multiyear ice, 10

NAUI, 79
neoprene, 21, 22, 25, 27, 28, 34
    boots, 27
    closed-cell, 22
    crushed, 22
    drysuit, 22, 27, 29
    gloves, 28
    hoods, 27, 28
    mitts, 28
    seals, 22, 25, 34
    wetsuit, 21
nylon, 22, 23, 31, 35, 39

O-rings, 36
open-cell foam, 31, 65
overhead ice, 1, 16, 21, 54, 66
oxygen, 14, 16, 42, 66, 67

pack ice, 10, 11, 46
pancake ice, 10, 11
personal flotation device, 42, 43
personnel, 2, 14, 15, 17, 42, 46, 48, 49, 50, 51, 52, 55, 57, 62, 63
    rescue, 42
    surface, 15, 17, 42, 46, 48, 49, 55, 57, 62, 63
PFD. *See* personal flotation device.
pitons, 43, 61
planning, 1, 2, 14, 50-52, 66
polar ice, 10
polypropylene, 30, 39, 40, 41, 42
pressure ridges, 46

Qualofil, 42

radiant barrier, 31
regulator, 2, 3, 35, 36-37, 58
    backup, 2, 35, 37, 58
    double-hose, 2, 3, 36
    environmental kits, 36
    free flow, 37, 58
    freeze up, 37, 58
    keeping water out of, 37
    primary, 2, 35, 37, 58

single-hose, 2, 13, 36
valves, 13, 36, 37, 58
rescue, 16, 19, 39, 64, 66, 67, 69
    divers, 39
    operations, 69
    personnel, 42
    procedures, 66
research diving, 2, 79
reverse stratification, 4
rivers, 8, 10
rope bag, 41, 54
rubber, 23, 24, 25, 27, 29, 35, 36
    boots, 27
    cap, 36
    drysuit, 23, 24, 35
    latex, 25
    mitts, 27
    natural, 23, 25
    rings, 27, 29
    silicone, 25
    synthetic, 23
    vulcanized, 23, 24, 35
rule of thirds, 54

safety, 1, 2, 13, 14, 15, 16, 18, 33, 39-42, 43, 45, 46, 48, 49, 50, 51, 52, 54, 55, 57-67, 69, 79
    checks, 18
    diver, 14, 16, 48, 50, 51, 54, 59, 60, 61, 67
    equipment, 39-42
    harness, 13, 14, 33, 39-40, 41, 45, 52, 58
    hole, 49
    lines, 13, 39, 40, 41, 43, 45, 50, 59
    officer, 79
    procedures, 15, 57-67
    stop, 54, 55, 57
scientific divers, ix, 3, 39, 79
screw, 13, 14, 41, 43, 47, 49, 61
scuba, ix, 2, 13, 32, 36, 39, 53, 58
sea ice, 10, 11
    floes, 10, 12
seals, 16, 17, 22, 23, 25, 26, 27, 28, 30, 33, 34, 35, 52, 59, 60
    drysuit, 25, 26, 27, 28, 34
    failure, 60
    gloves, 27, 52
    latex, 22, 23, 25, 26, 27, 28, 33, 34
    neck, 16, 22, 23, 25, 27, 33, 34, 60
    neoprene, 22, 25, 34
    replacement, 34
    silicone, 25
    wrist, 16, 22, 23, 25, 28, 30, 34, 59
shell suits, 23, 29, 42
shelter, 2, 13, 14, 17, 46, 55, 58, 67
shovel, 14, 42, 43, 47, 49, 50
Siberia, 4

single-hose regulators, 2, 13, 36
sled, 43, 48
snow blindness, 14, 62
snow ice, 9
snowmobile, 43, 45, 52
spokes, 49, 50
spring turnover, 4
standby diver, 41, 59, 60, 61
stratification, 4, 5, 14
    reverse, 4
strobe lights, 13, 50, 57, 61
    flashers, 13, 61
    flashing, 50, 57
sunburn, 14, 62
sunglasses, 42, 62
surface-supplied diving, 19, 39
synthetic pile, 30

temperatures, 1, 2, 4, 8, 36, 37, 38, 43, 62, 63, 79
    air, 4, 8, 36, 37, 38, 62, 63
    water, 1, 2, 4, 36, 63, 79
tender, 1, 14, 16, 17, 18, 29, 39, 40, 42, 43, 46, 49, 50, 52, 53, 54, 55, 58, 59, 60, 62, 67
    communication with, 16, 18, 39, 50, 52, 53, 58, 59, 60
    duties and responsibilities of, 14, 29, 39, 46, 49, 50, 52, 53, 54, 55, 56, 59, 62, 67
    equipment, 14, 42, 50
    line-pull signals, 14, 16, 18, 39, 40, 50, 51, 52, 53, 54, 59
    surface, 1, 17, 39, 43, 46, 58, 60, 67
    thermal protection, 42, 50
tether lines, 14, 50, 52, 53, 59, 60, 66
thermoclines, 4, 9
Thinsulate, 31, 42, 65
Thintech, 42
toboggan, 43, 48
training, vii, ix, 1, 2, 13-19, 21, 39, 52, 65
    altitude diving, 52
    confined-water, 16
    drysuit, 13, 16, 21
    ice-diving, 13-19
        advanced, 19
        open-water, 17-19
    surface-supplied diving, 39
trilaminate, 23, 24

Ultrex, 42
undergarments, 14, 16, 21, 22, 23, 27, 29-32, 34, 65
    fleece, 30
    heated, 31, 32
    open-cell foam, 31, 65
    radiant barrier, 31
    synthetic pile, 30

Thinsulate, 31, 65
woolly bear, 30, 65
unisuit, 2, 3
upwelling, 6, 9

valves, 13, 14, 15, 17, 23, 26, 27, 31, 33, 34, 35-36, 37, 38, 52, 53, 58, 59
    cylinder, 35-36, 37, 38, 52, 58
    exhaust, 17, 23, 26, 27, 31, 59
    inflator, 15, 17, 26, 31, 33, 34, 53, 58, 59
    H, 35
    K, 35
    regulator, 13, 36, 37, 58
    Y, 35
visibility, 1, 9, 15, 39, 49, 53, 55, 57, 58, 60
    Antarctic, 58
    freshwater, 9
    ice diving, 1, 9, 58
    lake, 9, 58
    low, 39, 58, 60
    plankton blooms, 58
    silty conditions, 53, 58
    snow cover, 49, 58
    thick ice, 58
vulcanized rubber drysuit, 23, 24, 35

water
    access to, 46
    accidental immersion, 43
    cold, vii, ix, 1-2, 4-10, 14, 21, 27, 36, 57, 63, 79
        environment, 4-10, 14
    column, 58, 60
    confined, 16
    contraction, 8
    density, 8
    entering, 53
    exercise in, 63
    exiting, 54, 55, 67
    expansion, 8
    freezing, 33, 36
    freshwater, 2, 4, 8-9, 14, 33, 37, 52
    inhalation of, 63
    intrusion, 28
    lake, 1, 4, 5, 6, 8, 9, 14, 58, 65, 79
    layers, 4, 6
    leaks, 35
    ocean, 4, 7
    open, 13, 17, 33, 52, 66
    physics of, 14
    salinity, 10
    saltwater, 8, 14
    seawater, 10
    shallow, 59, 60

soapy, 34, 35
surface, 4, 6, 8
temperatures, 1, 2, 4, 36, 63, 79
visibility, 1, 9, 15, 39, 49, 53, 55, 57, 58, 60
volume, 8
warm, 4, 7, 8, 9, 21, 52
waterproof, 16, 23, 25, 42, 48, 50
    boots, 42, 50
    clothing, 42, 48, 50
    gloves, 50
    overboots, 42
    suit, 16
    zipper, 23, 25
wax, 34
weather, 1, 8, 14, 21, 33, 37, 42, 50, 52, 54, 69
    cold, 1, 14, 21, 37, 69
    conditions, 42, 50, 54
    forecast, 14, 50
    freezing, 33
weight, 14, 17, 19, 22, 32-33, 46, 52, 55, 59, 65, 66, 67
    ankle, 33
    belt, 15, 19, 33, 52, 55, 59, 65, 66, 67
    release, 17, 33, 66
    systems, 14, 32-33
weight belt, 15, 19, 32, 33, 52, 55, 59, 65, 66, 67
    dropped, 19, 33, 59
    lost, 15, 59, 65
    release, 66
wetsuits, 2, 3, 16, 21, 22, 27, 31, 66
    hoods, 27
    neoprene, 21, 22
wind, 4, 6, 8, 10, 11, 15, 21, 42, 46, 50, 57, 58, 62
windburn, 62
wind chill, 14, 62
windproof, 58
woolly bear, 30, 65

Y line, 50
Y valve, 35

zipper, 17, 23, 24, 25, 33, 34, 35, 60
    care and maintenance, 33, 34
    failure, 60
    guard, 25
    leaks, 60
    length, 23, 24
    location, 24
        back, 23, 24
        diagonal, 24
        horizontal, 24
    lubrication, 17
    waterproof, 23, 25

About the Author

John Heine is an experienced scientific and recreational diver. He has dived in many areas of the world, including both poles and tropical areas in between.

Heine, who became a NAUI Instructor in 1980 and an Instructor Trainer and Course Director in 1982, is a certified Ice Diving Specialty Instructor. Having conducted many leadership-level training programs for NAUI, he was awarded NAUI's Outstanding Service Award in 1992 and elected into the NAUI Hall of Honor in 2014.

He earned a B.S. in biological sciences from the University of California at Irvine and a master's degree in marine science from the Moss Landing Marine Laboratories of the California State University. He is a past president of the American Academy of Underwater Sciences (AAUS).

Heine, who has conducted many scientific and sport dives under the ice, spent 10 seasons in Antarctica doing research dives through ice that was 10 feet (3 meters) thick, in water temperatures of 28.6°F (-1.9 °C) and air temperatures as low as -20°F (-29°C). He has also done cold water and ice diving in Alaska and in lakes in the Rocky Mountains. He has served as a member of the diving control board for the National Science Foundation, Office of Polar Programs.

Heine, an accomplished writer and photographer, has published scientific articles in journals such as the *Journal of Phycology, Journal of Experimental Marine Biology and Ecology, Marine Ecology Progress Series, Polar Biology,* and *Journal of Chemical Ecology.* His diving-related publications include books about advanced diving technology and techniques and drysuit diving for NAUI, *Scientific Blue-Water Diving* for the California Sea Grant Program, *Scientific Diving Techniques* published by Best Publishing, and articles or chapters in the proceedings of the American Academy of Underwater Sciences, *NOAA Diving Manual, Sources: The Journal of Underwater Education,* and *Underwater USA.* His underwater photographs have appeared in catalogs, textbooks, magazines, educational programs, and on websites. He is a past contributing editor for *Sources.*

Heine works as the diving safety officer for the National Science Foundation Division of Polar Programs and as the editor of *CalCOFI Reports,* a marine science journal supported by the Scripps Institution of Oceanography, NOAA, and the California Department of Fish and Wildlife.

www.ingramcontent.com/pod-product-compliance
Lightning Source LLC
Chambersburg PA
CBHW040251170426
43191CB00018B/2379